Very Best
To The "Girls"
The Royal Eye
Hospital Of
Manchester

John T. Flynn

Strabismus

A Neurodevelopmental Approach

Nature's Experiment

With 63 Illustrations

Springer-Verlag
New York Berlin Heidelberg London
Paris Tokyo Hong Kong Barcelona

John T. Flynn, M.D.
Professor of Ophthalmology
Bascom Palmer Eye Institute
University of Miami School of Medicine
Miami, Florida 33101
USA

Library of Congress Cataloging-in-Publication Data
Flynn, John T., 1931–
    Strabismus: a neurodevelopmental approach: nature's experiment /
John T. Flynn.
        p. cm.
    Includes bibliographical references.
    Includes index.
    ISBN 0-387-97409-1 (alk. paper).—ISBN 3-540-97409-1 (alk.
paper)
        1. Strabismus—Etiology.   2. Strabismus—Pathophysiology.
I. Title.
        [DNLM: 1. Strabismus.   WW 415 F648s]
RE771.F58   1991
617.7'62—dc20
DNLM/DLC
for Library of Congress   90-10140

Printed on acid-free paper.

Typeset by Publishers Service of Montana, Bozeman, Montana.
Printed and bound by Edwards Brothers, Inc., Ann Arbor, Michigan.
Printed in the United States of America.

9 8 7 6 5 4 3 2 1

ISBN 0-387-97409-1 Springer-Verlag New York Berlin Heidelberg
ISBN 3-540-97409-1 Springer-Verlag Berlin Heidelberg New York

*To the many, many infants and children with strabismus
it has been my privilege to help along the way,
this book is dedicated with love, admiration, and respect.*

Preface

Over the more than three decades of my life as a physician, I have been constantly amazed at how subtle and elegant nature is as a teacher. Our questions to her, though, must be clear and unambiguous. Otherwise, the answers we receive are likely to be misleading and confusing. As I have matured as a clinician, I have tried to improve my questions to increase my chances of receiving an answer. For the past decade, I have been pondering the subject of strabismus with which I have busied myself for practically two and one-half decades. I began to realize that my time, my share of wisdom, my abilities to carry out the prodigious work necessary to create a book out of nothing but thought, reading, and reflection on the work of others, as well as my own experience, were perhaps becoming limited. I do not doubt that they will become even more limited! Thus I have been led to write this book. Further, I am left in greater awe of prolific writers, particularly those who write with the precision and attention to detail necessary for a medical text.

Let me warn the reader at the outset that my approach in this book is "teleological." I am well aware of the conflict between science's notion of causality as only local and instrumental as opposed to the anthropomorphic notion of purpose or design in nature implied by the choice of this teleology. I chose this approach, however, because I am convinced that strabismus is, in fact, not some hodge-podge assembly of unrelated sensory and motor phenomena without a common material basis, but rather a very clear expression of a design flaw in the formation of the visual nervous system. Careful and scrupulous study of the phenomenology of strabismus on many levels would lead us to a fruitful conception of the nature of this misdesign and hence to a more basic knowledge of the visual system's normal design. In this sense, strabismus is for me one of nature's most wondrous experiments. Its study will answer many questions about the formation and development of the visual nervous system, questions we cannot answer by other means. Hence, teleology for me means specifically looking for evidence of design in strabismus.

In a wider perspective, I see this effort in the sense best expressed by Goethe in his letter to Frau von Stein, "I became aware of the essence of form with which nature, as it were, always toying and experimenting, brings forth the infinite varieties of life."

When I came to write this book I chose to abandon the time-honored (and to me somewhat time-worn) method of referencing every point made in the development of thoughts and arguments. Rather than interrupt the narrative flow with exhaustive references (which always tempt me, as the reader, to look them up to see if, in fact, they support the author's premise—a temptation, I confess I yield to more frequently now than in the past), I have chosen to use an annotated bibliography listing the sources I consulted in developing my thoughts. I invite the reader to consult these sources and read my comments on them at any point in the book—at the end of each chapter or in the narrative itself when I have not been clear. To provide the reader with a further safeguard against egregious error on my part, many of my friends in the clinical and basic sciences have read and critiqued the chapters specific to their areas of expertise. They are truly my collaborators in this endeavor and I am greatly indebted to each of them. None of them are coauthors for they did not write the chapters nor are they responsible for my conclusions. All of them, however, have inspired me through their work and I am grateful for their wise counsel in shaping my thinking on the various topics in the book.

There is another group I would like to acknowledge—my beloved colleagues at the Bascom Palmer Eye Institute. Edward W. D. Norton, my Chairman, Bob Lingua, my friend and co-worker in the Children's Clinic, and the men and women of our faculty generously provided me with support and encouragement in this effort, even when it meant more work for them. I am blessed to work in that special place in American ophthalmology, the Bascom Palmer Eye Institute. There is no other like it.

On another level, Dr. Carl Kupfer and his staff at the National Eye Institute, especially Dr. Constance Atwell and Mr. Ed McManus, have provided a great deal of support. Dr. Donald Lindberg, Mr. Jim Cain, and the staff at the National Library of Medicine have provided me with a "home" in which to work, the most stimulating library of its kind in the world. The National Library of Medicine I have come to value as truly a national treasure.

Finally, without the many hours of work devoted to this project by my beloved wife, Roseanne, who has accompanied me on many of my life's mad pursuits (at least they must appear so to her), and by my patient secretary, Mr. Frank Wilson, this book would never have made it past the early stages of its gestation. To them also, I am deeply indebted.

It is my fondest hope that this little book will in some small way serve to draw attention to strabismus as an entity that serves us, students of the visual sciences, as an inverted telescope, enabling us to look back to when the visual system was very tiny, very fragile, and yet very highly organized, as it needed to be for its role as the queen of our senses. Further, if this book entices some bright young minds to think thoughts they might never have, and to visualize ways to help those many wonderful children with strabismus, who are the inspiration for this book, it will have succeeded beyond measure for me.

John T. Flynn
Bethesda, Maryland

Contents

1
Why Write This Book?

The search for truth is in one way very difficult and in another very easy, for it is obvious that no man can master it fully nor miss it wholly, but each adds to our knowledge of nature and from the facts all assembled, there arises a certain grandeur.

Aristotle

If I may be permitted the luxury of beginning a book by sharing its purpose and contents with the reader, I take that luxury gladly. My topic, strabismus, has fascinated and perplexed me (among many others) for over a quarter of a century. Often in despair of ever understanding anything about the topic, I have put aside inquiry into the many questions patients present when I examine them and have resorted to a mechanical way of thinking about the condition that persists in its worst form as the sterile dogmatism— "if the eyes are in turn them out, and if they are out turn them in." But my demon will not go away. And so it is that I come to write this book.

I also take a further luxury to tell the reader what this book is not. It is not a book written to solve the many clinical management dilemmas presented by the patient with strabismus. This is not a clinical management text. There are many of these authored by superb clinicians who perform this task far better than I. Rather, my purpose is to propose a theory grounded in the developing anatomy and function of the nervous system and to ask as many questions within the framework of that theory as well as our modern knowledge of the nervous system, the answers to which might establish, beneath the practice of our art, a science.

The inspiration for this effort arose from reading a biography of David Hilbert, the great German mathematician whose life spanned the late 19th and early 20th centuries. At the turn of this century, he gave the inaugural address at the International Mathematical Society meeting held in Paris, France. The title of this dissertation was "Mathematische Probleme," and in it he surveyed the field and its accomplishments during the 19th century. But he used those very accomplishments as a beacon for the future. He proposed some 23 questions or problems derived from primarily the work of 19th-century mathematicians. The solutions to these have encompassed the history of modern 20th-century mathematics. I do not pretend to play a role in my discipline similar to Hilbert's. He was truly a giant

1

in that science which was mature as he spoke. As he said in that provocative essay, "If we would obtain an idea of the probable developments of (mathematical) knowledge in the immediate future, we must let the unsettled questions pass before our minds." And so I come to the major purpose of this book: to let pass before our minds, the reader as well as myself, major problems (questions) in strabismus, the answers to which will, it is my hope, enhance our art and perhaps provide a footing for its claim to be a science.

In writing this book I am also aware of Newton's famous dictum, "Hypothese non fingo." The hypothesis I put forward, though, contains no mysterious forces or factors to which Newton took exception. It is grounded in the ontogenesis of the nervous system. Within that context, strabismus is seen as an anomalous development of that system. This central hypothesis lends itself to testable questions on several levels. Anatomy, physiology, clinical phenomenology and symptomatology, and behavior are a few. Like all hypotheses, it is only as good as the last question of its validity answered successfully. As the philosopher of science Karl Popper believes, we can only falsify a theory, never prove it true. If indeed it is an incorrect formulation of strabismus, the efforts expended to prove it wrong will not have been in vain, but rather, will give rise to better and more viable hypotheses about our subject. I labor this point because I am aware that visual scientists of world renown feel that no theories in strabismus are worth the name. Though this attitude appears well placed, any science, if it is to be worthy of the name, proceeds by two routes, theory and experimentation. If we are not to be mired endlessly gathering observations and "facts" about strabismus with neither an inherent logic to relate the facts nor a plan that suggests how and where to look for them, then we best proceed by proposing and critically testing a hypothesis. The former method (which very much describes, in my viewpoint, what we do in strabismus today) leads to a form of scientific inductivism, the sterile millienarianism of Bacon, which was aptly critiqued by Medewar: "Sciences which remain at Bacon's level of development," he pointed out, "amount to little more than academic play." The latter method, proposing testable hypotheses, might be described as the Galilean method and led directly to a revolution in the physical sciences and later to the biological revolution of today. Galileo clearly recognized the necessity of formulating the experimental method with us today: the deliberate manipulation of physical objects for the purpose of testing a clearly stated prediction of a hypothesis. This act of creative imagination was in itself far removed from the machinelike operations of the inductive, fact-gathering approach of Bacon. It is the one I propose for our journey.

If the reader should choose to join me, we will proceed in these chapters to follow a path that seems logical to me. We will propose a question about a specific topic, for example, how do we get a visual system? Here we will treat the neurogenesis and histogenesis of the visuomotor system. This chapter will give rise to the next: What might an injury or insult to that nervous system do? From these two we will proceed to the central question of concern in this book: What is strabismus? This chapter will explicitly state my central hypothesis. I will try to remain aware of the slippery slope that is the nature of hypothesis generation and remember the other explanations of the phenomena described. My goal is to seek critical tests that distinguish between these alternative explanations.

By now, I hope the reader has noted that I refer to strabismus as a visuomotor anomaly and I will continue to do so throughout this text. The reason is to keep ever in mind the dual nature of strabismus. We would not experience the phenomenon of vision as we humans do unless both parts of the system functioned as one. This whole approach was aptly expressed for me in another context by von Monakow: "we see with our whole brains."

Proceeding further with the task at hand, we will bring such varied disciplines as visual psychophysics, development of vision in the infant, overall development of the infant, neural imaging of the central nervous system, and neuropathology to bear on our central topic, strabismus.

It is this process, then, that I hope will give us the tools and the verifiable facts with which to build a framework. And it is within such a framework that we will acquire knowledge on this fascinating visuomotor developmental anomaly. And so I invite the reader to accompany me on a journey in my mind—a thought experiment in my cherished field of endeavor, strabismus.

2
What Is the Neural Substrate
of Strabismus?

Nobody would attempt to define within any practical amount of space, the general concept of analogy which dominates our interpretation of vision . . . It is not at all unlikely that it is futile to look for a precise logical concept, that is, for a verbal description of the visual analogy. It is possible that the connection pattern of the visual brain itself is the simplest logical explanation or definition of this principle.

John von Neumann

To view strabismus from what I believe is the correct perspective, we must examine, in some detail, its neural substrate. Though this is not a textbook of developmental neurobiology, much of importance in our inquiry comes directly from this field. We will divide the task into several parts and cover the principles and some details of the embryogenesis of the visual nervous system: its neurogenesis (formation of neurons), histogenesis (formation of the various tissues that constitute the visual nervous system), and synaptogenesis (formation of connections between various parts of the visual nervous system), which give rise, en ensemble, to organogenesis (formation of the afferent and efferent visual systems). Stressed are principles and wherever possible, as examples of those principles, aspects of the development of the visual system so that the reader can become familiar with both the principles of nervous system development and the expression of these principles in the visuomotor system.

Developmental Mechanisms

Principles

Certain generalizations emerge from a study of the development of the central nervous system (CNS). The first of these is that the CNS is, throughout its phylogenetic and ontogenetic history, an epithelium, a tissue that exists in sheets and in which cells are stabilized through close apposition with one another with scant intercellular material, in contrast to a mesenchyme with loosely packed cells and abundant intercellular material. A second generalization is that within this epithelium most cells are generated at sites other than those they occupy in the mature tissue. The final generalization is that each event in the elaborately integrated spatial and temporal program of development reflects the interplay of genetic and epigenetic factors. A given cell is endowed with a repertoire of possible responses; the particular response is determined by its environment.

The differences in position, shape, and final form that the epithelium of the CNS takes are the result of the sequential and historical interaction of a number of driving forces and regulatory elements. The driving forces are cell division, cell migration, and cell death. The regulatory processes, acting in ever-changing concert with these driving forces at different stages of development, are cell adhesion (synapse formation) and cell specialization and differentiation. Consideration of these cellular processes under the single heading of "topobiology" (a comprehensive hypothesis to account for the evolution and development of animal form) by Gerald Edelman provides a framework within which to begin to understand this complex event. If a given cell within this epithelial matrix is genetically endowed with a repertoire of possible responses from which a particular response is determined by its environment, then a corollary is that once a critical step in development is taken, be it genetically or epigenetically induced, normal or abnormal, a consistent series of subsequent steps is set in motion. A normal or a mutant gene may, for example, exert a single direct effect on a given cell population and each emerging property of the cell's system in turn provides the setting for a series of subsequent events and the emergence of new properties. The story of the miswiring that occurs in the afferent visual system as a result of the albino gene is a striking example of this causal chain. Understood in this context, the final form is a product of both its genes and environmental factors—epigenetic events.

Time

To organize our knowledge further, it is necessary to delineate the time at which events occur and view the events from a perspective made specific for us through examples relevant to the developing visual system. It is obvious that the CNS is a dynamic system with much overlap in development of its different parts. Thus, while the neural tube is closing at the anterior neuropore rostrally, primary neurogenesis is occurring in the region of the brain stem caudally. All events are related to a single variable, time. This is and will remain the axis of development throughout (Table 2.1).

Morphogenesis

In its broadest categorization, human development can be broken down into five periods, four of which occur prior to birth.

TABLE 2.1. Human central nervous system ontogenesis.

Weeks of gestation	Event
0–2	Three germ layers, neural plate, and groove develop
3	Optic vesicles appear
5	Cerebral vesicles, choroid plexi, and dorsal root ganglia develop
8	Differentiation of cerebral cortex begins; meninges form; cerebral spinal fluid circulation is present
10–20	Corpus callosum develops; major fissures of the cerebral cortex develop
21–25	Neuronal proliferation in the cerebral cortex ends
28–40	Secondary and tertiary sulci form; synaptogenesis occurs in the cortex
40+	Glial cell production and myelin formation occur

Adapted, with permission, from Sidman RL, Rakic P. Development of the human central nervous system. In: Haymaker W, Adams RD, eds. Histology and Histopathology of the Nervous System, 1982:3–145. Courtesy of Charles C Thomas Publisher, Springfield, Illinois.

I. Preimplantation development (week 1): After successful fertilization, subsequent cell divisions form the blastomere of the cleavage state, the morula (mulberry), and eventually the blastocyst, which contains two distinct cell types: the trophoblasts, which will go on to form the placenta, and the *inner cell* mass, which is the precursor of the embryo proper.

II. Early implantation (weeks 2 to 3): By the end of the first week of development, the embryo has implanted in the wall of the uterus. During gastrulation in weeks 2 and 3, three embryonic layers are formed: ectoderm, mesoderm, and endoderm. *Neurulation* begins with formation of the neural plate and subsequent formation of a closed neural tube.

III. Embryonic development (weeks 4 to 8): The most important events during embryonic development are major folding of the embryo and the initial formation of all organ systems. *Developmental insults at this stage result in major congenital defects* (Figure 2.1).

IV. Fetal development (weeks 9 to 38): Growth and maturation of existing structures are the hallmarks of fetal development. Minor malformations can be induced; the optic and central nervous system are the organs at greatest risk for injury during this period of development.

V. Postnatal development (weeks 38 to 2+ years): In the visual system, maturation of the visual cortex and peristriate cortex and myelination of the afferent and efferent fiber tracts take place.

The earliest event of concern is neurogenesis, which begins in the third week with the formation of the neural plate and continues through the period of myelination and formation and functioning of synapses necessary for development of the normal binocular visuomotor system. For convenience in organizing knowledge, I have tabulated, for each site in the visual system, the times at which the neurons that will give rise to the functions of interest are born, migrate, and begin synapse formation (Table 2.2).

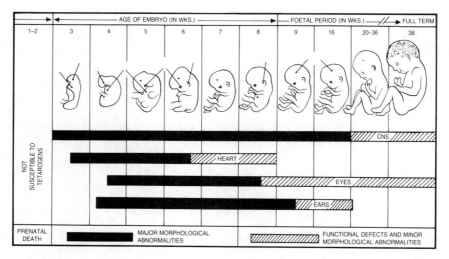

FIGURE 2.1. Timetable and events in human development with periods of maximum sensitivity to teratogenic effects. Modified, with permission, from Moore KL. *The Developing Human: Clinically Oriented Embryology.* 3rd ed. Philadelphia: WB Saunders; 1982.

Processes

Although the human central nervous system must be, in its form and function, one of the most complex instruments in the universe, its structure may be understood in terms of four fundamental and overlapping processes and their integration (Figure 2.2). Each process is finite and tightly time-locked to a developmental plan that has begun to emerge from recent studies on different parts of the system.

Neurogenesis

The generation of neurons begins, for the entire central nervous system, in the ventricular zone surrounding the ventricles (Figure 2.3), 2 weeks postconception, with a few neuroblasts and continues unabated at the rate of about two to three cycles per 24 hours, until about 20 weeks postconception, after which there is no further evidence that neurons are generated in the nervous system. During the process some 10^{12} neurons are produced in all. Their birth dates, although not firmly known in all cases, reflect an overall pattern controlling the maturation of various parts of the visual nervous system.

Migration

After their birth in the ventricular zone, neurons migrate to distant sites where they become functional. The process is almost universal in the nervous system;

TABLE 2.2. Visual system neurones: Developmental timetable.[a]

Cell population	Birth (weeks)	Migration (weeks)[b]	Synaptogenesis (weeks)	Myelination (months)[c]	Function
Retina	5–14	7–? (except photoreceptors and retinal pigment epithelium)	12–20	8–14 (except postlaminal axons)	Light transduction, primary visual processing
Lateral geniculate nucleus					
Magno	8–?	10–30	12–30	10–15	Further visual processing
Parvo	10–?				
Visual cortex primary (VI)	12–?	6–16+	12–?	10+	Further visual processing
Associative (V2, V3, V4, ...)	12+–?	?	12–?	10+	Motion system or color, form system
Superior colliculus	10–?	?	10–20	7–14	Eye movements in response to processed visual signal
Cranial nerves					
III	6	6–10	?	5	Eye movements in response to visual signal
IV	6	6–10	?	5	
VI	7	7–10	?	5	
Pontine and vestibular nuclei	7	7–10	8–12	5	Supranuclear integration of eye movements
Pontine paramedian reticular formation	?	?	?	7–30+	

[a] Various sources.
[b] Weeks postconception.
[c] Months postconception.

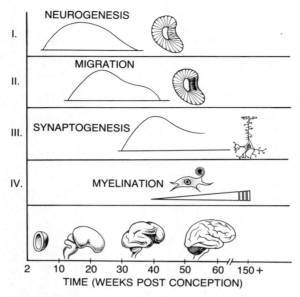

FIGURE 2.2. The four processes concerned with nervous system development—neurogenesis, migration, synaptogenesis, and myelination—with a timetable indicating when these processes occur.

however, exceptions do occur. For example, the retinal pigment epithelium and the layer of retinal receptors, generated in the outer and inner layers, respectively, of the optic cup, remain in place next to the extension of the ventricular cavity, where they are formed. The latter becomes the potential subretinal space between the layers.

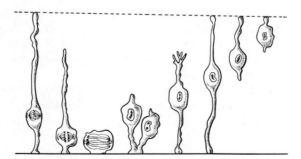

FIGURE 2.3. Birth of neurons in the subventricular tissues. Modified, with permission, from Sidman RL, Rakic P. Development of the human central nervous system. In: Haymaker W, Adams RD, eds. *Histology and Histopathology of the Nervous System* 1982: 3–145. Courtesy of Charles C Thomas Publisher, Springfield, Illinois.

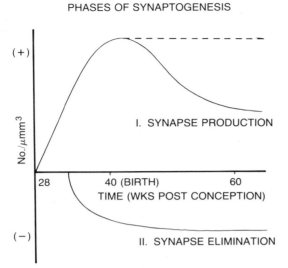

PHASES OF SYNAPTOGENESIS

FIGURE 2.4. The process of synaptogenesis if biphasic: synapse production and synapse elimination. The final number of synapses is a product of the balance between the two.

Synaptogenesis

Neurons do not form synapses until they arrive at or near their final destination. The process of synaptogenesis is critical in determining the final form and function of the developing brain. The process seems to consist of two phases: synapse generation, in which many more connections between cells than will ultimately be necessary are formed initially, and synapse elimination, a process of remodeling in which those connections that will be functional are selected to survive and the remainder are eliminated (Figure 2.4).

For example, very early in the formation of the cortex, the region of the cerebral wall immediately beneath the pial surface layer of cortex containing primitive neurones, is subdivided into a marginal zone immediately beneath the pia and a subplate layer by the formation of the future cortical plate (Figure 2.5). The latter contains no cells early in development. The mantle and subplate layer form a rich plexus of synapses among themselves and with incoming thalamic axons. The process is the same throughout the cortex—primary sensory, motor, or associative. Most of these primitive synapses disappear with time and, indeed, the subplate layer itself totally disappears later in cortical ontogenesis. Yet it plays a critical and central role early in development, perhaps in specifying the final position and connections of the ingrowing thalamic axons.

This phenomenon in which a tissue arises in development, flourishes for a period, and then disappears is a recurring theme in CNS ontogenesis and is reminiscent of the development of the primary vitreous, tunica vasculosa lentis, and optic stalk in the eye.

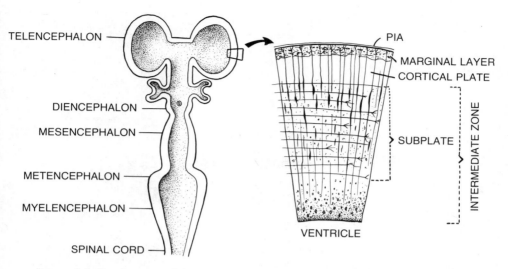

FIGURE 2.5. Development of the marginal layer of the cortex subdivided into mantle and subplate layers separated by the empty future cortical plate. From Chun JJM, Shatz CJ. A fibronectin-like molecule is present in the developing cat cerebral cortex and is correlated with subplate neurons. Reproduced from *The Journal of Cell Biology*, 1988; 106:857–872 by copyright permission of The Rockefeller University Press.

Myelination

Myelination in the CNS is produced by the oligodendrocyte. Long sensory and motor fiber systems become myelinated early; the late appearance of the myelin sheath in interconnecting systems of the brain, association fibers, and the like could be related to the acquisition of task specification and speed of conduction. Both of these properties might be critical to the acquisition of learning, memory, and other intellectual abilities (Figure 2.6).

Defects in myelination do occur and, early in life, present as degenerative disorders, for example, the leukodystrophies, (metachromatic, adrenophilic, and sudanophilic). These devasting diseases of infancy and early childhood are inborn metabolic insults to the lipoprotein myelin. All result in early CNS degeneration and death.

To summarize, four developmental processes—neurogenesis, migration, synapse formation and elimination, and myelination are essential in providing the form underlying the function of the CNS, in general, and our structure of interest, the visuomotor brain, in particular. They are processes that operate in a very complex and still, in part, obscure manner to translate the information contained in the one-dimensional genetic code into the three-dimensional tissue, the human brain. Our next task is to look at the result of these processes as they give rise to the form of the human brain.

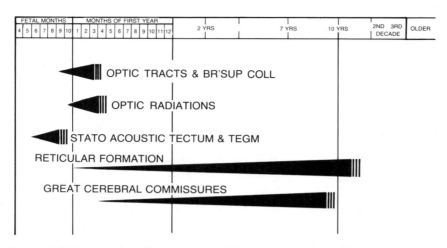

FIGURE 2.6. Process of myelination in several important segments of the central nervous system. Redrawn, with permission, from Yakovlev PI, Lecours AR. The myelogenetic cycles of regional maturation of the brain. In: Minkowski A, ed. *Regional Development of the Brain in Early Life*. Oxford: Blackwell Scientific; 1967:3–70.

Development of Structure

Neural Induction: Development of the Neural Plate and Neural Tube

The earliest embryonic organ, the chorda mesoderm, interacts with the overlying ectoderm to initiate formation of the nervous system. It is likely that the forebrain is induced by prechordal mesoderm, whereas the brain stem and spinal cord are induced by the notochord (Figure 2.7). In humans, closure of the neural tube occurs at about the 22nd day at the level of the cervical cord; the tube then becomes rapidly zippered dorsally in both rostral and caudal directions, with final closure of the anterior and posterior neuropores occurring during the 4th week postconception. Differential growth of the tube gives rise to its "M" shape because of the cephalic, pontine, and cervical flexures delimiting major areas of the brain (Figure 2.8). Defects here are major, for example, anencephaly and cyclopia, and are far removed from our area of interest.

Neurogenesis

The epithelial sheets that line the now closed neural tube rapidly replicate and become organized into a pseudostratified epithelium. Cell numbers increase logarithmically at the rate of about two to three generations per day. Repeated cell division is accompanied by the development of a rounded cell body during

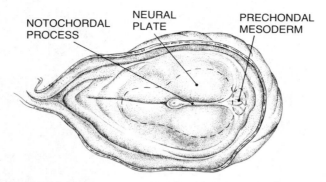

NOTOCHORDAL PROCESS   NEURAL PLATE   PRECHONDAL MESODERM

FIGURE 2.7. Induction of the neural tube destined to become the forebrain by the prechordal mesoderm and the brain stem and spinal chord by the notochord. Modified, with permission from Moore KL. *The Developing Human: Clinically Oriented Embryology.* 4th ed. Philadelphia: WB Saunders; 1988.

mitoses and is followed by the extension of cytoplasmic processes anchoring the cell to the ventricular surface and the outer limiting membrane of the CNS (Figure 2.9).

These changes in cell position produce the marginal, intermediate, subventricular, and ventricular zones in early neurogenesis. Radial glial cells, though their origins are more obscure, probably originate early from the ventricular zone.

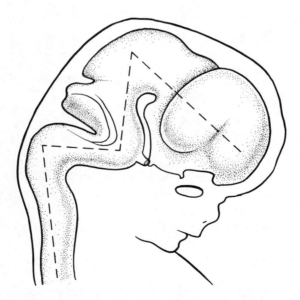

FIGURE 2.8. Early definition of the major brain area by means of the cephalic pontine and cervical flexures. Redrawn, with permission, from O'Rahilly R, Gardner E. Z Anat Enwicklungsgesgh, 1971; 134:8, by permission of Springer-Verlag.

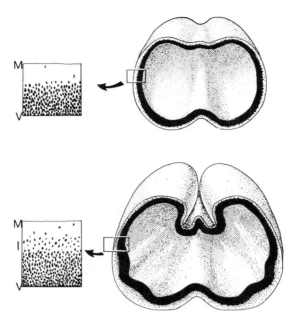

FIGURE 2.9. This cross section of the neural tube at the level of the telencephalon illustrates the process of neurogenesis producing the marginal (M), intermediate (I), and subventricular and ventricular (V) zones. Adapted, with permission, from Sidman RL, Rakic P. Development of the human central nervous system. In: Haymaker W, Adams RD, eds. *Histology and Histopathology of the Nervous System* 1982:3–145. Courtesy of Charles C Thomas Publisher, Springfield, Illinois.

The interplay between the two—the neurons and the glial cells of the CNS—is critical at the next stage, cell migration.

General Form of the Brain at 4 to 11 Weeks of Gestation

The primordium of the optic vessels can be recognized at this stage; their stalks are fused in the midline at the site of the future chiasm (Figure 2.10). The ventral systems of the neural tube, including the hypothalamus, the mesencephalon with the mesencephalic nuclei, and the brain stem motor nuclei, all develop earlier than the dorsal sensory nuclei. By the fifth week the neurons of the motor nuclei

▶

FIGURE 2.10. Gross morphology of the human brain during neurogenesis. Modified, with permission, from Sidman RL, Rakic P. Development of the human central nervous system. In: Haymaker W, Adams RD, eds. *Histology and Histopathology of the Nervous System* 1982:3–145. Courtesy of Charles C Thomas Publisher, Springfield, Illinois.

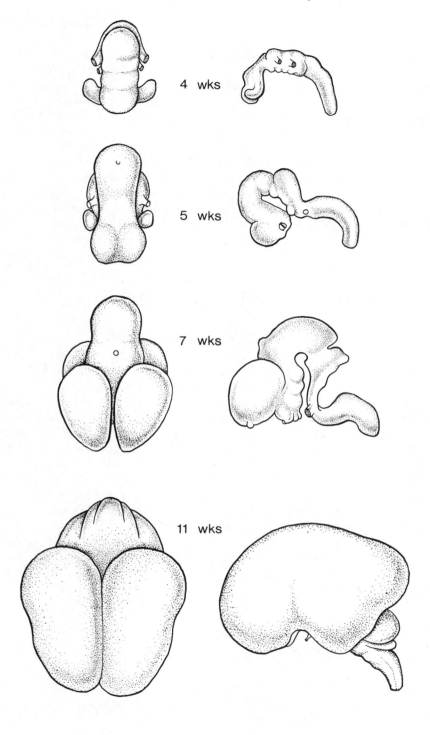

4 wks

5 wks

7 wks

11 wks

of cranial nerves III, VI, and XII emit axons ventral to the neuraxis, and in the ventromedial cell columns, neurons that include cranial nerve IV, V, and VII to XI nuclei can be recognized. Their axons pass dorsally and laterally through the visceral motor nuclei to emerge from the lateral wall of the brain stem, except for cranial nerve IV, which emerges dorsally. The primary afferents of the sensory ganglia associated with the brain stem and spinal cord are differentiated and enter the neuraxis as cranial nerves V and VII and the vestibular portions of VIII, IX, and X at this stage. Cranial nerve VIII is already sending efferent axons to the contralateral otocyst.

By the seventh and eighth weeks, the medial longitudinal fasciculus and the major cerebellar and tectobulbar tracts, as well as the principle neuronal systems for brain stem reflex activity, are in position. The first extraocular muscles can be observed in utero ultrasonographically at 8 weeks. During the sixth week the cerebral hemispheres balloon outward from the dorsolateral wall of the telencephalon. Earlier, when the telencephalon is larger than the lateral ventricles, the dorsal wall is composed of only a cell-rich ventricular surface and a cell-poor marginal layer.

Internal and External Configuration of the Brain (12 Weeks to Term)

During the next 28 weeks, there is extensive elaboration of the neural tissue constituting the cortical plate of the telencephalon. The growth of the structure is so rapid that the expanding cerebral hemispheres come to cover the diencephalon (optic vesicles), the mesencephalon (oculomotor and trochlear nerves), and the metencephalon (pons and sixth cranial nerve) (Figure 2.11). During the third month, the cerebral wall thickens by threefold, as a result of ingrowth of fibers from the thalamic nuclei. Generation of new cortical cells expands the surface area of the cortex and increases cortical thickness itself. The increase in cortical surface area plays a role in the creation of fissures, gyri, and sulcii. This does not completely explain these formations, however, as decompression of the intracranial space or removal of the gray matter overlying the white matter does not alter or diminish the pattern of gyration. At 11 to 12 weeks the first fissure, the sylvian, appears. At 6 months the central sulcus develops. Otherwise, the cortex remains smooth (as an adult lissencephalic cortex). At 6.5 months the calcarine and callosomarginal fissures appear. Although all fissures and gyri of the human brain can be recognized at birth, many are shallow and poorly demarcated. They do not attain the final external topography of the adult brain until approximately 12 years after birth.

Development of the Telencephalon

Because its scope encompasses much of importance to the visuomotor system, we treat the development of the telecephalon as a whole. On pragmatic grounds let us use the structure of the cortex as it forms as our pattern for classification.

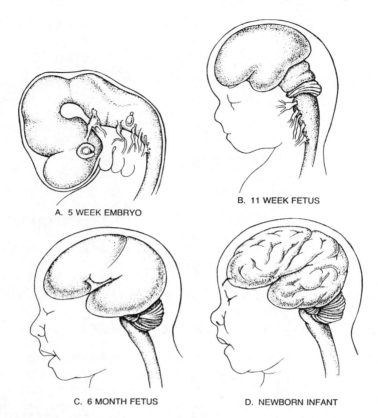

A. 5 WEEK EMBRYO

B. 11 WEEK FETUS

C. 6 MONTH FETUS

D. NEWBORN INFANT

FIGURE 2.11. External changes in the brain from 5 to 40 weeks. (A) 5-week embryo, (B) 11-week fetus, (C) 6-month fetus, (D) newborn infant. Modified, with permission, from Noback, CR (illustrator: Demarest RJ). The Human Nervous System: Basic Elements of Structure and Function, New York: McGraw-Hill, Inc., 1967.

During the fifth week of gestation, the future cerebral hemispheres are represented as lateral evaginations of the prosencephalon, forming two thin-walled chambers (see Figures 2.9 and 2.10). The basal and basolateral parts will become the basal ganglia and related structures. The dorsal part of each hemispheric vesicle remains thinned at this early stage and consists of a ventricular zone, an intermediate zone, and a marginal zone, which later will become the site of the future cortical plate.

The divisions of the cerebral cortex are those of Rakic (as modified from Filimanov):

1. Neocortex: These are the cortical territories having all of the cardinal developmental layers—ventricular zone, subventricular zone, intermediate zone, cortical plate, and marginal zone. The subdivisions of the cortex are characterized by heterotypical architecture in the primary motor and sensory receptive cortices (that is, the calcarine cortex of area 17) or homotypical cortex, more usual of the associative cortices.

2. Allocortex: The allocortex contains an incomplete set of cardinal developmental layers, including the following:
   a. Archicortex: subiculum, hippocampus, and dentate gyrus
   b. Paleocortex: prepyriform, olfactory tubercle and bulb, septal and diagonal areas
3. Mesocortex: The mesocortex is the transitional zone between the allocortex and the neocortex.

Development of the Neocortex

At an early ontogenetic stage the cerebral cortex lacks a cortical plate. Prior to 6 weeks the wall consists of a ventricular zone and a thin marginal zone. Between 6 and 7 weeks an intermediate layer develops as a result of the appearance of cells between the ventricular and marginal zones. Cells of the subventricular zone make their appearance as well. During fetal week 7, newly postmitotic ventricular cells migrate outward to form a new layer at the junction of the intermediate and marginal zones, and thus begins the formation of the neocortical plate. Schematically, the development can be summarized into five stages (after Rakic):

Stage I. Initial Formation of the Cortical Plate (Fetal Weeks 7 to 10)

During the sixth and seventh fetal weeks of gestation the formation of an intermediate layer is initiated when cells of the ventricular zone of the cerebral vesicles into the intermediate zone forming the preplate outward (Figure 2.12). By the end of the seventh week these young neurons move across the intermediate zone and begin to form an incipient cortical plate. It is interesting that during this stage, the first synapses forming lie in the most superficial laminae above the incipient cortical plate and in the subplate zone immediately below the future cortical plate but not in the plate itself. During weeks 9 and 10 the intermediate zone becomes clearly divided into an inner zone of closely packed cells (the so-called subplate layer) and an outer marginal zone containing numerous fibers but few cell bodies.

Stage II. Primary Condensation of the Cortical Plate (10 to 11 Fetal Weeks)

During the 10th and 11th fetal weeks, the cortical plate progressively thickens, becomes more compact, and is clearly demarcated from the intermediate zone. By the 11th week, the first major wave of migration across the intermediate layer is finished. Directly beneath the cortical plate, the subplate layer is acquiring more fibers from the ascending axons of thalamic neurons. The number of these afferent axons will greatly increase during the next few weeks. The times of arrival and the precise spatial patterns of the terminals of these arriving afferent axons may actually play a role in determining the corresponding dendritic patterns adopted by the target neurons.

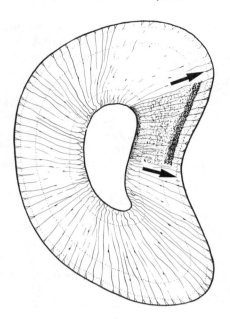

FIGURE 2.12. Formation of the cortical plate: future cortical neurons migrate through the intermediate layer, pausing in the subplate layer (darkened) before invading the cortical plate. Modified, with permission, from Sidman RL, Rakic P. Development of the human central nervous system. In: Haymaker W, Adams RD, eds. *Histology and Histopathology of the Nervous System* 1982:3–145. Courtesy of Charles C Thomas Publisher, Springfield, Illinois.

Stage III. Bilaminate Plate (Fetal Weeks 11 to 14)

The uniform and compact cortical plate observed in the second stage further subdivides during approximately the 11th to 13th weeks into an inner zone occupied mainly by cells with relatively large nuclei and an outer zone of cells with densely packed oval nuclei elongated along the axis perpendicular to the cortical surface.

This heterogeneity results from the partial maturation of the deep-lying cells that arrived during the earlier stage and a new wave of somata of immature cells that take up a more superficial position in the cortical plate. This is the pattern of migration that gives rise to the so-called "inside out" positioning of cells in the cortical plate; that is, the earlier-arriving neurons take up positions in the lower cortical laminae (V and VI), whereas the later-generated younger cortical neurons take up positions in the upper cortical laminae (II and III).

Stage IV. Secondary Condensation (Fetal Weeks 13 to 15)

During the 13th to 15th weeks of gestation, the ventricular zone becomes progressively thinner as a larger percentage of the cells generated there move outward and fewer cells per unit volume continue to divide. The subventricular zone remains relatively wide and cell rich. The cortical plate at this stage becomes homogenous in appearance and resembles a thickened version of the plate of stage II. Most of the young neurons in this stage are enlarging though they still remain elongated and in a relatively compact arrangement. The cell bodies destined for the prospective middle layers have arrived by this time. Few neurons are entering the cortical plate so it is sharply separated from the underlying subplate zone. This interpretation of a fluctuating morphology of the cortical plate implies phasic proliferative activity in the germinal zones or phasic migration of neuronal somas (probably both). The first wave forms the primary cortical plate (stage I) and subsides at the stage of condensation (stage II). The second major wave begins with cell proliferation in the ventricular and subventricular zones, probably during stage II, and continues through the stage of the bilaminate cortex (stage III) to the stage of secondary condensation (stage IV).

After the final mitotic division in the ventricular zone, postmitotic cells enter the intermediate zone and assume an elongate bipolar form oriented toward the cortical plate. Throughout a pathway of some 3500 micrometers or longer across the intermediate zone, the migrating cells are closely apposed to elongate, radially oriented glial processes that, at this stage, span the full thickness of the cerebral wall. These radial glial fibers constitute guidelines that facilitate cell migration through the maze of closely packed cell processes and cell bodies that compose the telencephalic wall at the late stages of cortical development. Several generations of postmitotic cells migrate successively along the same radial fibers and become stacked in a common vertical column within the cortical plate, the somas of the more mature cells lying deeper than those of the less mature ones. This vertical columnar organization is very pronounced during stage III of cortical development; only later does it become obscured by the growth of lateral dendrites and other horizontal and oblique processes.

Stage V. Prolonged Maturation (Synaptogenesis and Myelination,
Fetal Weeks 17 to Second Postnatal Year)

This stage of cortical maturation lasts from the 17th fetal week well into the postnatal period. A very wide range of interrelated developmental events take place during this prolonged crucial period. By the fifth lunar month (20th week), neuron precursors are few to be seen in the reduced ventricular zone of the cerebral hemisphere. Neurons that were generated prior to the 16th week are still migrating and have yet to reach the cortical plate. The subventricular zone continues to serve as a germinal area, providing an increasing number and variety of glial cells. By the end of the 5th month, the cell somas of the middle zone of the cortical plate become more widely separated from one another than cells in the outermost and innermost zones so that the cortical plate assumes a three-layer form. The middle zone represents future mature cortical layer 5. Its pyramidal cells are already developing numerous dendritic branches. The more superficial cell somas are less mature, whereas many of the newly generated cell somas still in transit have yet to migrate through deeper layers and become properly aligned in their cortical laminae. During the 5th and 6th months, subpopulations of pyramidal and fusiform neurons become distinguishable among the neurons of the middle zone. In general, dendritic spines are the last components to develop. In humans, the spines appear first on the large pyramid neurons of the fifth layer by the seventh lunar month and only after birth are they formed on the dendritic processes of smaller neocortical neurons. These morphological features merit more detailed attention as expressions of developmental disease (see Chapters 3 and 4).

By the seventh lunar month the cortex is divided into six layers. Lamina 1 has relatively few cell bodies and is sharply demarcated from the underlying layers. The superficial third of the cortical plate is divided into an outer zone of densely packed cell bodies (lamina 2) and a wider, looser interzone (lamina 3). These layers remain very immature until after birth. Between lamina 3 and the pyramidal cell zone (lamina 5) is a densely populated wide zone of small cells that will become lamina 4. On the deep side of the pyramidal zone is a loosely bound zone (lamina 6) that merges with the underlying fiber layer (future white matter).

Stellate cells become recognizable in the seventh lunar month. These differ from pyramidal and fusiform neurons in possessing processes that are confined to the general vicinity of the cell body. It seems that the more complex the dendritic and axonal structure of the stellate cells, particularly those cells found in layer 3, the higher their evolutionary rank.

The six layer pattern present in the fetal cortex is not strictly homologous to the laminae of the adult neocortex. For example, some cell somas in layer 4 at the seventh fetal month will be distributed in layers 3, 4, and 5 in the adult. Moreover, many young neurons still reside within the subplate zone during the last trimester and even after birth. Generation of neocortical neurons ceases during the last few months of gestation. The outer marginal layer of the neocortex contains a special class of horizontally-oriented large neurons called Cajal-Retzius cells. The dendritic bouquets of all pyramidal neurons are anchored to the processes of these cells. They disappear during the first half of the first postnatal year in humans. Another fascinating contemporary component of the marginal zone is the transient subpial layer, the so-called superficial granular layer of Ranke. This layer has been recognized only in humans. During the 13th and 14th fetal weeks it is present as a thin condensation of cells visible at the external surface of the cerebral cortex. The absence of mitotic figures in the layer leads to the conclusion that the cells multiply exclusively at their fountainhead in the subventricular tissues of the prepyriform area of the archicortex at the base of the telencephalic vesicles and then migrate tangentially along the external surface of the vesicles. They form functional synapses and later disappear, though it is not clear how.

Regional Differences in the Telencephalon

Three general principles govern regional differences in the telencephalon:

1. Within a given region of cortex, neurons of the deeper layers arise and differentiate earlier than superficial neurons. Those with long axons achieve maturity before all others.
2. Among the different regions, the neurons earliest to mature are those in the specific projection areas that receive direct, compact, precisely patterned afferents from the thalamic nuclei and send long axons to the subcortical formations.

3. The cortical areas that are more diffusely connected with subcortical regions and have abundant cortical association fibers show considerably more prolonged periods of neuronal development.

Projection Systems in the Telencephalon

Area 17 is distinguishable from its adjacent cortical areas at 5 months of gestation on the basis of its more diffuse cell population in the marginal lamina. Other layers are first seen in area 17 during the sixth lunar month and only thereafter in areas 18 and 19. The differentiation of layers in 18 and 19 progresses at a slower pace in these latter areas during the remaining months of gestation. Myelination in the geniculocalcarine tract begins during the 10th lunar month. The development of synaptic contacts proceeds over a period of many months until well beyond birth both in humans and in animals.

Association Systems

The earliest commissural system to cross the midline between the two cerebral hemispheres is the anterior commissure, which can be first identified at 10 weeks of gestational age. By the 12th week the corpus callosum has crossed the midline just anterior to the hippocampal commissure. Malformations in the region of the lamina reuniens lead to agenesis of the corpus callosum.

Development of the Diencephalon

Ventral Diencephalon

The diencephalon has conventionally been regarded as a transitional zone between the telencephalon rostrally and the caudal neuraxis of the CNS. The diencephalon and telencephalon, unlike other regions, are thought to be induced in common by the prechordal mesoderm and, as a result, come to share many interconnections. At 3 weeks of gestational age, the lateral walls of the open neural tube at the diencephalic level take the shape of two broad and shallow concavities, which are the incipient optic vesicles. They are connected across the midline by the torus opticus. Cyclopia and the earlier severe faciotelencephalic malformations in which a midline unpaired eye develops can arise from a defect either in the underlying prechordal mesoderm or in the early telencephalic or diencephalic structures, at any time up to and including this stage when the paired optic vesicles are discernible. Development of the optic vesicle is one of the major morphogenetic events of the fourth week of gestation. It dominates diencephalic development throughout the early period of gestation. Early in the fourth week the optic vesicle begins to indent, its first step in conversion into a cup. Under the influence of the vesicle, the overlying ectoderm forms the incipient lens plate. The sector of the vesicle wall adjacent to the surface ectoderm is destined to form the neural retina; on the other

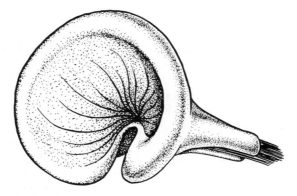

FIGURE 2.13. Invaginating optic cup, with the fetal fissure invaded by optic nerve axons. Modified, with permission, from Sidman RL, Rakic P. Development of the human central nervous system. In: Haymaker W, Adams RD, eds. *Histology and Histopathology of the Nervous System* 1982:3–145. Courtesy of Charles C Thomas Publisher, Springfield, Illinois.

side of the vesicle wall is the pigment epithelium. By the sixth week, the neural retina has reached its adult dimension of about 0.2 mm, whereas the pigment epithelium remains permanently a single layer of cells. Late in the fourth week the vesicle invaginates to form the optic cup, a crucial feature of which is the optic fetal fissure (Figure 2.13).

This fissure results from a second invagination in the form of a groove running from the hollow of the developing cup lengthwise across its ventral aspect. The ventricular cavity between the developing neural retina and the pigment epithelium remains open and in contact via this optic stalk with the third ventricle of the diencephalon itself. The neural retina, which separates the internal ventricular space from the external space of the fetal fissure, is continuous with a similarly positioned tissue in the optic stalk. The neural retina is composed of a ventricular and a marginal zone, with the mitotic figures occurring, as always, at the ventricular surface. When the cells are postmitotic the somas will migrate to the opposite side, that is, toward the marginal zone. In one respect, the formation of an intermediate zone between the ventricular and marginal zones, the developing human retina resembles other sectors of the embryonic brain wall. In another it differs, being "outside in" in its organization: ganglion cells first followed by cones with the last of the ganglion cells and amacrines. Rods are generated late. Soon afterward, the postmitotic neurons generate axons that pass into the marginal zone at the vitreal surface of the retina. These axons course in sequence along the vitreal surface into the fetal fissure on the ventral external aspect of the optic stalk and onto the ventral surface of the diencephalon at the level of the future optic chiasm. They then pass along the external surface of the diencephalon toward the eventual position of the lateral geniculate bodies.

During the fifth week and early part of the sixth week of gestation, tissues at the opposed margins of the fetal fissure fuse, neural retina fuses to neural retina, and pigment epithelium fuses to pigment epithelium so that the site where the original retinal axons had passed from the vitreal surface into the fetal fissure, now enclosed within this structure, becomes recognized as the familiar optic disc. As the retina continues to grow, more nerve fibers form and fasciculate with the pioneer fibers to increase the cross-sectional area of the optic nerve head. Axon bundles expand in that part of the fetal fissure running ventrally along the optic stalk and the bundle comes to form the optic nerve, "overshadowing" both the ventricular cavity and the germinal tissues that lie in the stalk. These germinal tissues in the stalk give rise to the glial cells which form the septa of the optic nerve. Within the neural retina itself, five major classes of neurons are generated in overlapping sequence. From earliest to latest these are the ganglion, cone, amacrine, horizontal, bipolar, and rod cells. The sequence begins in the central retina, which has already produced several classes of neurons when the ventral peripheral retina is just producing its initial class. The earliest differentiating ganglion cells are recognizable by light microscopy during the fifth week of gestation. By the sixth week the somata of many ganglion cells have taken up position partly across the marginal layer. Amacrine cells are forming before the end of the 6th week and horizontal cells by the 9th week; by the 11th week, bipolar neurons and some photoreceptors are differentiating. Most cone photoreceptors differentiate earlier than rods. By the seventh lunar month the retina appears mature except for the relative narrowness of the inner plexiform layer, where synapses form between the ganglion, amacrine, and bipolar cells. Development of the macula is still incomplete and the transient layer of Cheivitz is present. During the seventh and eighth months, the outer segments of the photoreceptor cells develop and the organism is able to respond to light.

Dorsal Diencephalon (Lateral Geniculate Nucleus)

At about the 11th week of gestation, the two sides of the thalamus fuse in the midline, eliminating a part of the third ventricle and forming the massa intermedia. Although the neuron population within the thalamus is still homogenous in appearance, several fiber systems connecting the thalamus to other regions have already begun to develop. During the seventh week, bundles of pioneer axons pass between the thalamus and the telencephalic vesicles. The origin and direction of these axons are unknown, but it is almost certain that at least some of these early fibers are destined to become thalamocortical projections. Axons of retinal ganglion cells likewise grow around the lateral surface of the diencephalon to produce the optic tract by the seventh week. By the eighth week, the lateral geniculate nuclei are demarcated from the generally homogenous thalamic cell mass. From their site of generation at the lumen of the third ventricle, geniculate neurons migrate to the lateral and dorsal walls of the diencephalon, to form an initially homogenous cell layer. The earliest cells generated are those that will furnish the magnocellular layers of the mature nucleus. Lamination begins to appear in the structure when it is invaded by incoming optic tract axons. The process of lamination is completed in the lateral geniculate body by 22 weeks. Massive development of the pulvinar nucleus during the fifth to seventh months of gestation displaces the lateral geniculate nucleus from its dorsal position to a more basal position. This dramatic growth of the pulvinar (a possible source of input to the oculomotor system for pursuit eye movements) takes place after the fourth month. Prior to this development, the ventricular germinal zone lining the third ventricle, which is the source of pulvinar neurons, has been quiescent for weeks.

An overview of thalamic development indicates that the first components to differentiate are the specific sensory nuclei subserving the visual, auditory, tactile, and postural and sense modalities (the lateral and medial geniculate nuclei, the ventral basal complex, the ventral lateral nuclei, and the ventral anterior nuclei, respectively). The limbic nuclei develop in relation to the mammillary bodies. The nonspecific thalamic nuclei and midline nuclei develop rather early relative to their hypothalamic and thalamostriatal connections. The last to differentiate are the so-called association nuclei. Myelination of the thalamic parts of the optic tract begins in the ninth month. The visual radiation myelinates at the tenth lunar month, the auditory radiation soon after birth, and the somatosensory radiation in the ninth lunar month.

Development of the Posterior Neuraxis (Mesencephalon and Pons)

Mesencephalon

The mesencephalon develops from the fifth neuromere, which lies directly above the rostral terminus of the notochord. The vague rostral margin of this neuromere permits no clear division between the mesencephalon and the diencephalon. By contrast, a relatively sharp ventral sulcus at the caudal border of the fifth neuromere demarcates the mesencephalon from the pons (the isthmus). During the second lunar month, the mesencephalon encloses a huge chamber called the mesocoele of the mesencephalic ventricle. At the beginning of the second month, an intermediate zone appears in the basal half of the mesencephalon but only later in the alar half. By the third lunar month the anatomy, both surface and internal, has so altered that many anatomists object to the terms *basal* and *alar* and would substitute *tegmental* and *tectal* instead. The first component to be recognized in the tegmental or basal intermediate zone is the primordium of the oculomotor nucleus. Its earliest postmitotic cells (3 weeks) promptly emit axons that emerge at the base of the mesencephalon. Through the eighth fetal week, the right and left oculomotor primordia show no continuity across the midline. In the ninth week, the right and left nuclei become united across the midline by the formation of the prospective nucleus of Perlia. Somewhat later, in the 10th and 11th weeks, appear midline cells that migrate to form the cell mass of the Edinger-Westphal nuclei. All components of the oculomotor nuclei are recognizable by the end of the third fetal month. Cells of the underlying red nucleus and other mesencephalic structures differentiate during the second and third fetal months.

Still another special feature of the developing mesencephalon is the remarkable growth of its altar (tectal) plate during the second and third months. This plate thickens bilaterally so that a median longitudinal depression along the narrow roof plate separates the two sides. Later, a transverse depression comes to separate the rostral from the caudal part. In this way four bulges form the incipient quadrigeminal plate representing the future right and left superior and inferior colliculi. Growth of this quadrigeminal plate is impeded rostrally by the already formed posterior commissure and the expanding cerebral hemisphere. Caudally, the plate comes to override the still undeveloped cerebellar anlage. Growth and thickness of the colliculi result mainly from the genesis of neurons in the ventricular zone, with passage of the somas of their cell bodies outward toward the external surface of the mesencephalon. Fibers of the human optic tract are clearly visible in the superior colliculus at the end of the second lunar month, and a cortex-like alignment of cell bodies in columns is recognized in the superior colliculus. The auditory system's lateral lemniscus reaches the inferior colliculus at approximately the same time. The brachium of the superior colliculus reaches the medial geniculate body during the third lunar month. Myelination in all structures of the mesencephalon precedes that in the diencephalon and telencephalon.

Rhombencephalic Isthmus

The isthmus is the ring of neural tissue constituting the wall at the rostral end of the rhombencephalon bordering the mesencephalon. Neurons of the trochlear nucleus are first seen in this structure during the second month. Axons from the trochlear nucleus decussate and exit the isthmus dorsally rather than ventrally. The reason is unknown.

Rhombencephalon (Pons and Medulla)

During the third to fifth fetal weeks, cranial nerve nuclei, including those of the sixth cranial nerve, become clearly visible in the intermediate zone of the pons.

Myelination in the Human Central Nervous System

Myelination in the CNS is produced by the oligodendrocyte. Long sensory and motor fiber systems become myelinated early; later, myelin sheath appears in the interconnecting systems of the brain itself, the association fibers, thought to be related to the acquisition of learning memory and other intellectual abilities.

In summary, we have taken a brief trip in space and time through the development of the nervous system particularly as it relates to the visual nervous system. The complexity of the events unfolding and the integration of many, many parts and many, many schedules of development are staggering. One has but to lightly peruse the literature on neuroembryology, particularly the neuro-embryology of the visual system, to be aware of this and also to be aware of the strides that are being made in understanding how the machinery is put together. It is conceivable that within the foreseeable future we will realize the truth of von Neumann's intuition of many years ago and come to understand vision through an understanding of the connections of the visual brain. More specific to us is our task to understand strabismus through an understanding of the "miswiring" of the visual brain.

3
What Might an Insult to that Nervous System Do?

Human organs respond to a large number of diverse dysmorphogenic influences with the production of a very limited repertoire of malformations.

John Opitz

In the last chapter we looked into the processes necessary to produce a central nervous system, more specifically, a visuomotor system. As with so many biological phenomena of seemingly staggering complexity and diversity at the end-product stage, these processes are built on simpler processes interacting within a tightly budgeted time span during development. For the central nervous system from the retina to the cortex and back on out through the oculomotor nerves, four processes occur: neurogenesis, migration, synaptogenesis, and myelination. From 2 to 90 weeks postconception (1 year after birth) most of the neurons of the visual system are generated and located in place, their synaptic connections are completed, and the myelin is laid down to make these connections task specific and the conduction via these connections rapid. The visual system of the infant during this period is astonishing in approaching (perhaps more rapidly than we dare guess) the adult in functional capacity.

In this chapter, I explore the general concept of insult or injury to that developmental process by which a visuomotor nervous system forms. The two areas on which I concentrate are genetic information and/or environmental factors as possible insults to the development of the nervous system.

Let us begin by viewing strabismus from a temporal perspective. It has been with us since at least the time of the papyri of ancient Egypt. It has, since antiquity, been seen as a stigma of inferiority—an idea that is troubling to the patient and difficult to dislodge from cultural folklore. The explanations sought for its occurrence range from old wives' tales of maternal shock or fright marking the infant to the mechanistic theory associated with the great name von Graefé, through the refraction theory again associated with another great name in our science, Donders, to the more contemporary theories of fusion by Worth, vergence innervation by Duane, and reflexogenic action by Chavasse. Strabismus constitutes an interesting historical walk through the pantheon of ophthalmology's greats and is beautifully detailed in Keiner's little book, *New Viewpoints on the Origin of Squint.* All, including the old wives' tales, contain more than a grain of truth. At the end of the last century in his address to the Societé Francaise d'Ophthalmolgie on the treatment of squint, Parinaud requested his colleagues to forget—even if for only a few hours—what they thought they knew about strabismus. In searching for the next pieces of the puzzle of strabismus, I feel myself in a position similar to Parinaud's.

Because the condition has been with us from antiquity and because there is evidence of little change or drift in its clinical appearance across races, geographic locations, and time, let us assume that we are dealing with a stable entity of very similar morphological features (external signs and symptoms). I hasten to add here, though, that there is a real need for large, population-based incidence (rate of occurrence of cases per thousand) and prevalence (total number of cases in a given population) studies. Although we all quote figures ranging from 1% to 4% or 5%, these badly need updating. The science of clinical epidemiology must be brought into the planning of such studies so that the data we gather will have the fullest possible meaning, both epidemiologically and clinically. The time spent prospectively organizing such studies with full collaboration between the clinician-scientist (for this is how I see us) and the epidemiological scientist will be well rewarded in terms of the value of the data gathered. Such a study appears to be underway in Israel and may represent a model for us. Such studies might reward us with clues to where next to look for specific risk factors for strabismus in populations, the next piece of the puzzle.

Let us now shift our focus from the population as a whole, with and without strabismus, to the unit in which strabismus has its origin, the fetomaternal relationship. Let us assume, for the moment, that the strabismus we see in our clinics today would be not very different from the strabismus of antiquity, and that if we could travel back in time and examine an infant or child with strabismus by the Nile River or between the Tigris and Euphrates rivers (even perhaps in the Riff Valley?), we would find that they all resemble very much our modern-day child. There would be many more similarities than differences and we, as clinicians, would instantly recognize strabismus in the children of the past as we do in the children of today. What does this tell us? That, in spite of enormous societal, cultural, environmental, medical, and other changes, literally leaping over civilizations and millennia, strabismus is a robust entity whose phenomenology has remained almost invariant with respect to time. And for me, it considerably narrows the focus of the search to a triad: the mother, the placenta, and the fetus. It thereby excludes the exotica and esoterica of today such as drugs, radiation, retroviruses, the Industrial Revolution, vegetarianism, flower power, and the like as being the necessary and sufficient cause(s) of strabismus, but does not exclude any or all of these as potential contributing causes. This may be self-evident to all (except me) but it is helpful to hold such a perspective when I think about the problem. I believe that the necessary cause(s) of strabismus lies within the mother, the child, and the placenta. As we shall see (Chapter 4), I will suggest that a specific temporal period (roughly the last trimester of pregnancy and the first 4 to 6 months of postnatal life) is critical to the genesis of strabismus. The

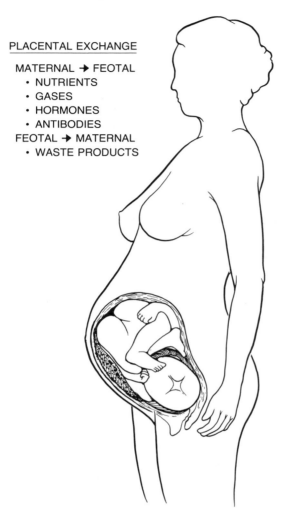

PLACENTAL EXCHANGE

MATERNAL → FEOTAL
 • NUTRIENTS
 • GASES
 • HORMONES
 • ANTIBODIES
FEOTAL → MATERNAL
 • WASTE PRODUCTS

FIGURE 3.1. The fetomaternal interface, the placenta, is critical to the structural development of the organs of the infant, including the central nervous system.

preparation for extrauterine life of the fetus entails enormous changes in the mother, the child, and their interface, the placenta. Let us briefly examine what is going on in each of our possible candidates experiencing the unique event:

1. Maternal changes during the third trimester
    Respiratory system
        Increase in tidal volume (40%)
        Decrease in carbon dioxide concentration
    Cardiovascular system
        Increase in cardiac output (30%)
        Increase in mean blood pressure

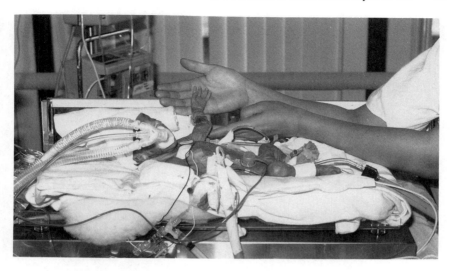

FIGURE 3.2. An infant of 24 weeks' gestational age on the typical life support systems necessary for extrauterine life.

Hormones
   Steroids (estrogen, progesterone, androgens): increase
   Human chorionic gonadotropin: stable
   Human chorionic somatotropin: decrease
2. Placenta
   Coupled with the enormous growth of the fetus, the placenta enlarges throughout most of the first two and one-half trimesters of pregnancy. During that time, in addition to being the site of gas, nutrient, electrolyte, hormone, antibody, and waste product exchange, the placenta also produces its own hormones (human chorionic gonadotropin, chorionic somatotropin, luteinizing hormone, thyrotropin, adrenocorticotropic hormone [ACTH], estrogen, progesterone, and probably testosterone (Figure 3.1). Parturition itself is thought to be triggered by a combination of oxytocin release by the maternal pituitary and fetal steroid hormone release by the fetal adrenal gland. Some or any of these may be potential agents: in particular, abnormal dosages of or times of exposure to the hormones constitute an insult to the developing nervous system of the fetus in the last trimester of pregnancy.
3. Fetus
   Although the changes that mother and the placenta undergo in the last 2 or 3 months of pregnancy are enormous, they are dwarfed by those occurring in the fetus. So many organ systems, from the nervous system to the integumentary system, begin to function to provide the fetus with support for life outside. One has but to pause beside an incubator containing a 24-week-old premature infant to realize the ghostlike similarity of this premature newborn to (Figure 3.2), and yet the appalling differences from, a normal newborn infant (Figure 3.3).

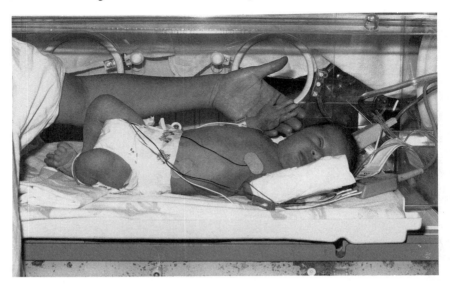

FIGURE 3.3. Normal 40-week-gestational-age infant requiring minimal life support.

The point I would make is that during this period of startling growth, the fetus doubles in weight in the last trimester, which is only a rough indicator of its maturation and readiness for extrauterine life. The major organ systems begin to operate while the fetus is making protein and fat, storing carbohydrate, and readying its own hormonal and immunological systems for the perilous trek to extrauterine life. With its very first breath, the fetus descends from a hypoxia equivalent to the top of Mt. Everest to sea level in terms of its blood oxygen. Cerebral, vascular, respiratory, and metabolic systems shift from a passive support to an active survival-oriented mode of function. It is in this maelstrom of change, probably second only to conception in terms of its dimensions, that the infant is born. We need to scrutinize this point in time and the events surrounding it, the events preceding it to about 7 months postconception, and, finally, those events 4 to 6 months postbirth for a potential source of the agent(s) of injury we seek. Development of the visuomotor nervous system is reaching one of its peaks during this period and, therefore, is particularly vulnerable to insult.

Let us summarize to this point. We began this chapter by looking at strabismus as a durable disorder that was present in antiquity and has changed, we suspect, very little over time; we know little about it epidemiologically, except that it affects about 1% to 4%–5% of children and occurs very early in life, but probably not at birth. This suggests the need to begin conducting well-designed population-based epidemiological studies to learn more about its habitus in different locales. There are tantalizing reports of differences in the incidence of convergent versus divergent deviations in Japan, Africa, the Middle East, Europe, and North and

South America. But more and better organized studies need to focus attention on who, when, where, and what before we can begin to suspect an answer to why.

Our next level of focus was on the fetomaternal relationship via the first human "interface," in the biological rather than in the computer sense, the placenta. The period on which we focused included the events of the last trimester in utero and the first two trimesters ex utero. In the last trimester, the mother begins to withdraw her life support systems and to change her physiological economy to suit that of a single person again. The fetus readies many of the critical life support systems it will need from its own armamentarium, and the placenta prepares to self-destruct, its usefulness coming to an end. (It is akin in this to many systems of interest to us, for example, the tunica of the lens, the primary vitreous, and the optic stalk; all live, flourish, and disappear, having served their most useful purposes. We learn more about this in the next chapter.) It is a time of growth and a time of decline, a time of birth and a time of death, a time of beginnings and a time of endings, to wax Dickensonian.

Now let us shift our focus to a still smaller scale, that of the gene and the molecule. Let us start with a simple question. Is it likely that strabismus is caused by a single genetic insult, a point mutation? I believe this is probably no more likely than the development of the central nervous system being under control of a single gene. It is more likely that thousands of genes are involved. But what of the data on concordant monozygotic twins versus discordant dizygotic twins? What of the data on families? All speak to the probability of n genes operating together with an unknown number of environmental factors. Monozygotes share all of the same genes; dizygotes share only 50%. The problem with the "genetic" interpretation of ordinary strabismus was well summarized by one observer: "the effect, strabismus, if it is a genetic effect, is far removed from its genetic cause." This does not by any means rule out a role, and an important role, in strabismus for genes. We have a clear-cut model in living organisms—the albino, be it an albino mouse, a Siamese cat, a "white" tiger, or an albino child. Miswiring of afferent visual system fibers, which begin at the retinal level and carry on up to the cortex, results in, among other effects, strabismus (Figure 3.4). Guillery, Hubel & Wiesel, Shatz and others have begun to detail the mechanisms by which this miswiring begins at the level of the optic stalk and continues on through the primary striate to peristriate cortices. Is a similar explanation likely in other cases of strabismus? If afferent fiber generation and routing were the problem, traces of it in the retina would have been detected by study of retinal function or retinal anatomy by generations of ophthalmologists examining and performing ophthalmoscopy on these children. Study of the retina leaves no doubt that something is very wrong with it in albinism. One has equally no doubt that nothing is wrong with the retina in ordinary strabismus. I would therefore come down on the negative side of this question and would not spend resources to look into the afferent visual system for the effects of the insult that might lead to strabismus.

One must nevertheless keep genes and the operation of genes very much in mind as a potential source of insult to the developing visual nervous system. But I believe we need to learn a good deal more about how they operate in combination, how

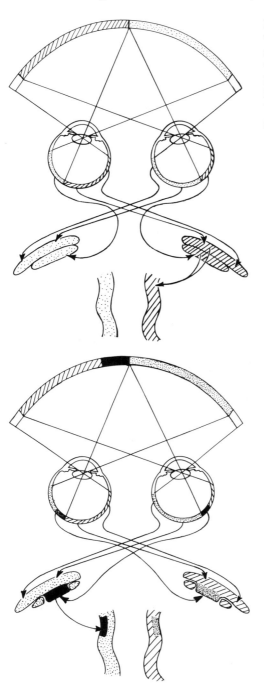

FIGURE 3.4. Schematic of the normal wiring of the afferent visual system and the miswiring of the afferent visual system in the albino cat. (A) Normal wiring. (B) Abnormal wiring. Derived from Guillery RW. Visual pathways in the albino. *Scientific American*, May 1974, p 45.

they are turned on and off, and in what sequences and numbers they occur before significant progress is made in the study of strabismus. It is not as simple and clearly defined a question as the molecular genetics of color vision or retinoblastoma has become because of the hard-won progress made in those fields of molecular biology.

I next turn attention to where I believe progress could be made (particularly in the production by neurobiologists of animal models), the application of the principles and most especially the thought processes of teratology to strabismus. I realize that for many, the jump from the usual conceptions of teratogens such as rubella virus, thalidomide, and maternal alcohol, and their dreadful effects on the fetus to strabismus is an enormous leap. Yet let us start simply: Teratology as a science is devoted to the study of the environmental contribution to abnormal prenatal growth and development. That is its definition. I am stretching the definition to include postnatal life because, I believe, the particular teratogens we might have in mind begin to act in utero and have their last effects in early postnatal life. This is so simply because it happens to be the time when the system is under development. Birth is truly an accident as far as some parts of the developmental timetable are concerned. Although interest in teratogenic agents began earlier, especially among such basic scientists as Hans Spemann and his students as exemplars of this school of experimental embryology, a substantial amount of information on teratogenic effects could be classified in medicine as folkloric prior to the 1950s and 1960s. It took the successive tragedies of thalidomide and rubella in those decades to rekindle serious interest in the subject.

Most of us are familiar with the context of teratogens as causes of major malformations and with the fact that these major malformations occur with the frequency of 2% to 3% in our population. It is fair to say, though, that at present, considerable debate still rages regarding the relative contribution of environmental teratogens to the causation of birth defects in our newborn population.

Granted that the preceding is true, I would nevertheless like to introduce a new frame of reference into our thinking about teratogens. I believe it is likely that a substance(s) that is during some part of neural development necessary to facilitate that development (Figure 3.5) but then continues to operate beyond its useful life span, is the immediate cause of strabismus in the central nervous system (Figure 3.6). This substance(s), which has a perfectly normal role to play in development, becomes, from this viewpoint, an environmental teratogen. As such, its action at a specific time results in the production of a series of developmental dysmorphologies, which give rise to the phenomena we recognize as the clinical syndromes of strabismus. I believe we can narrow our focus still further and say that the teratogen(s) at issue probably belongs to one of several classes of substances: (1) protein neural growth factors, which stimulate the growth of neuronal processes; (2) cell surface proteins which may serve as growth markers or guides to cell migration and synapse formation; (3) hormones and hormone-like substances, which serve as trophic support substances; or (4) the antagonists of these classes of substances, which bring the operation of any or all of them on

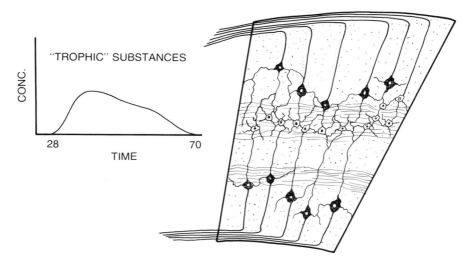

FIGURE 3.5. Normal operation of a trophic substance necessary for the development of normal synapses.

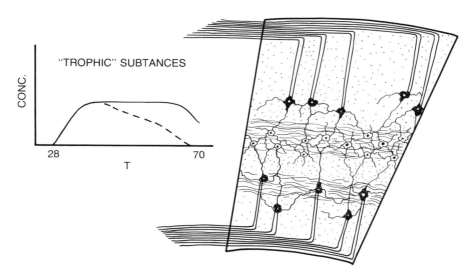

FIGURE 3.6. Prolonged action of a trophic substance, which results in abnormal development of central nervous system synapses and, hence, strabismus.

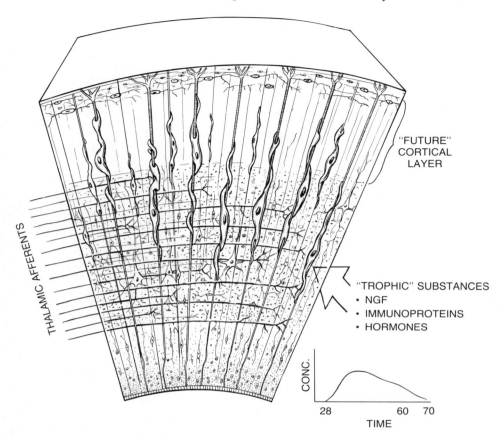

FIGURE 3.7. Operation of "trophic" substances necessary for normal synaptogenesis in the cortical subplate layer, a critical step in normal corticogenesis. NGF = nerve growth factor.

nervous tissue to a close (Figure 3.7). This list may seem very incomplete and far from specific in the eyes of developmental neurobiologists. But it seems to me to fit best with the concepts I hope to develop in this book. These substances are required for development of the nervous system during specific stages. As such, they must at some level be under the control of genetic factors, yet subject, I believe, to environmental influences as well. This concept is critical. These are agents that, at the right time and place, facilitate change and growth and development of the nervous system. But if their action(s) is prolonged, they become capable of producing specific dysmorphologies, one of which is strabismus.

Further, as a class, teratogens are known to act by a relatively limited number of pathogenetic processes. They may produce cell death, they may interfere with cellular differentiation or other basic morphogenetic processes, or they may

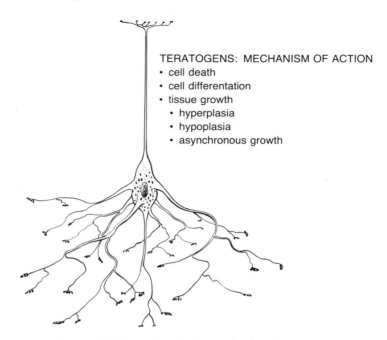

TERATOGENS: MECHANISM OF ACTION
- cell death
- cell differentation
- tissue growth
  - hyperplasia
  - hypoplasia
  - asynchronous growth

FIGURE 3.8. General mechanisms of action of teratogens.

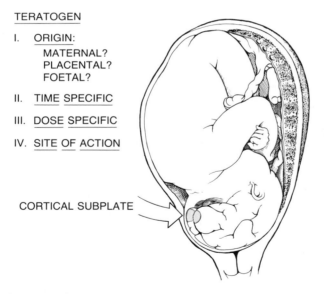

TERATOGEN

I.   ORIGIN:
        MATERNAL?
        PLACENTAL?
        FOETAL?

II. TIME SPECIFIC

III. DOSE SPECIFIC

IV. SITE OF ACTION

CORTICAL SUBPLATE

FIGURE 3.9. Summary of the action of a hypothetical teratogen on the developing central nervous system, resulting in strabismus.

alter tissue growth (hyperplasia, hypoplasia or asynchronous growth) (Figure 3.8). I believe it is by the last mechanism that our teratogen acts. As has been stressed throughout this chapter, the timing of the exposure, as well as its dose and host susceptibility (genetic?), is of critical importance in the operation of this teratogen(s).

In the model I propose, strabismus is a stable, dysmorphogenetic syndrome resulting from the operation of an extrinsic substance that is normally needed for nervous system development but becomes a teratogen only because its function should have, but has not, lapsed. The teratogenic effect is such that it is produced in the final stages of fetomaternal interaction (last trimester of pregnancy or early postnatal period) (Figure 3.9). The teratogen is one or a number of a small group of chemicals present in the nervous system of all fetuses (and likely to have been present in their nervous systems since humans have been in existence — it's "home baked"!). And its effects, probably more tightly time-specific than dose or host-specific, are what we identify clinically as strabismus. This then is in keeping with John Opitz's dictum with which we began this chapter.

4
What Is Strabismus?

He who sees things grow from their beginning will have the finest view of them.

Aristotle

I hope the reader has become aware, in the last two chapters, that a great amount of information has emerged in recent decades on the neurogenesis of the central nervous system in humans, other primates, and other animal species. In addition, in each of these species, specific timetables dictate the sequence in which events occur so that the whole system emerges as an orderly functioning unit at or around the time of birth. The timetable governing this process in humans is known with less precision than it is in other animals. But it is apparent that the effects of injuries to the developing nervous system in all species are very tightly bound to these timetables. It is against this background of central nervous system development and potential insult that I suggest we may begin to understand what strabismus is.

The Generic Model of Strabismus

Before going into the details of the hypothesis I am proposing to account for strabismus, let me digress to describe a generic model of strabismus that contains the elements I feel are common to every case seen in practice. I exclude from consideration here cases complicated by the occurrence of amblyopia, as that renders our thinking about the model unnecessarily complex and is not a direct concern of this book. First, the *time* of occurrence is in the first several years of life. Strabismus occurs, then, during the last stages of development of the visuo-motor system. It is unaccompanied by other major neurological disorders, so I exclude here as well from consideration the strabismus that accompanies cerebral palsy states and other major neurological disorders of the neonatal and infant period. That does not mean that strabismus is unaccompanied by other central nervous system developmental problems; rather, these other problems are more subtle and must be looked for in a different context than we are used to.

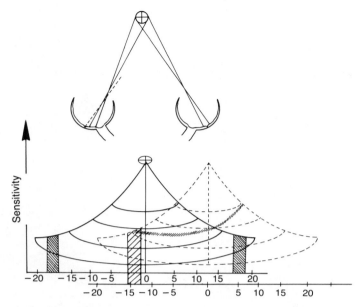

FIGURE 4.1. Binocular visual field misalignment in strabismus with the supression scotoma in the left, misaligned eye.

Second, the model of strabismus we employ presents three abnormalities of the visuomotor system that distinguish the strabismus state from any other motor or sensory anomaly it may superficially resemble. All three elements are considered to be present in every patient with strabismus if sought for. Conversely, they are never found together in any patient who does not have strabismus. The reason for this is, I believe, at the heart of the very nature of strabismus, but more on that later. A child then with our model of strabismus presents with the following:

1. An abnormal ocular posture such that the two foveas are not aligned on the same object of regard: As a consequence, the binocular visual field of the two eyes is out of register as well (Figure 4.1). The degree of the misalignment may vary from very small (1° or 2°) to very large (30° or more). The direction of the misalignment may be either convergent or divergent and it is, within limits, invariant with respect to which eye is fixing and which field of gaze the eyes are in. The important consequence of this state is that the foveas and the central visual fields of both eyes are out of register.

2. An inhibition of the visual information derived from the central visual field of the eye that is not fixating the target of interest: Depending on the circumstances in which it is measured, this takes the form of a suppression scotoma of variable depth up to 0.5 to 1.5 log units (see Figure 4.2 for normal comparison). Several characteristics distinguish this scotoma from any other pre- or postchiasmal visual field defect with which it might be compared. First, it alternates

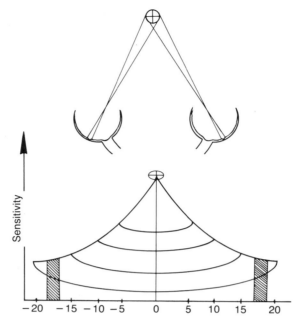

FIGURE 4.2. Profile of normal binocular visual field sensitivity (both eyes aligned).

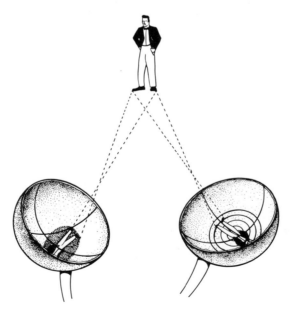

FIGURE 4.3. Areal extent of a suppression scotoma on the retina in strabismus (left eye deviated).

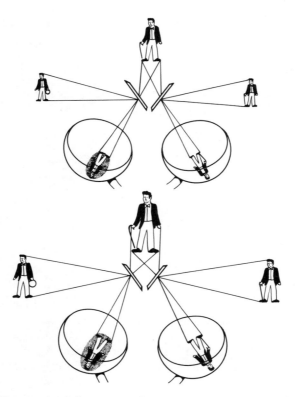

FIGURE 4.4. The extent of the scotoma in the central visual field of the strabismic increases in response to the use of a larger target.

freely between the two eyes and is found on some form of binocular perimetry only in the eye that is not fixating the target of interest. (Remember, we specifically excluded amblyopia earlier.) Under monocular testing conditions, it is absent. It has several other unusual characteristics as well. Although it is central and usually more extensive in the visual hemifield concordant with the direction of the deviation of the eye (that is, nasal retina suppressed in convergent deviations, temporal retina suppressed in divergent deviations), it extends beyond the vertical meridian horizontally, though it is limited in its vertical extent (Figure 4.3). When the scotoma is tested for by means of targets having similar contours projected in both eyes (so-called fusion targets), the *larger* the targets are, the larger the scotoma becomes (Figure 4.4). This is the reverse of the behavior of other scotomata in either the anterior or posterior visual system, where the smaller the targets are, the larger the scotoma becomes. Still another anomalous behavior can be detected within the scotoma; peripheral contours projected in the binocular visual field of both eyes can produce further suppression in the macular region of the deviated eye (Figure 4.5). These aber-

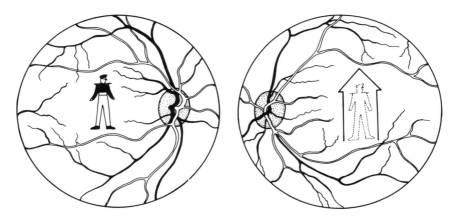

FIGURE 4.5. Influence of peripheral contours producing further suppression in the macular region of the deviated eye.

rant behaviors together with the fact, that for all practical purposes the scotoma, disappears completely when tested for under monocular conditions make this an exceedingly interesting and challenging neurological phenomenon.

3. Abnormal binocular localization of objects in space: Again, in our generic model, under binocular visual conditions, when a subject is tested for the localization of objects in space by the deviated eye compared with the fixing eye and against the well-understood rules of ocular projection (usually some technique must be employed to differentiate the visual fields of the eyes, such as red-green or striated glasses, crossed polaroid filters, or orthogonal afterimages, to bring the image of the object stimulating the deviated eye into consciousness), the localization of this visual object by the deviated eye is abnormal in a predictable direction, that is, toward alignment with the object fixated by the nondeviated eye (Figure 4.6). Though this phenomenon is doubted or trivialized by some, it is part of our model and part of the essential symptomatology of strabismus. Though its meaning may escape us, it is so prevalent a phenomenon that it must be encompassed within the framework of any theory of strabismus. Granted there are many frustrating and bedeviling aspects to this phenomenon, such as variability of the localization defect with the test employed to measure it or with the direction in which the eyes are pointing when it is measured. Yet these behaviors are, I submit, embedded in the very nature of strabismus itself and, correctly interpreted, are giving us important sensory and motor clues about the condition with which we are dealing.

These then are from my standpoint, that of a clinician, the characteristics that distinguish the strabismic state from all other patterns of abnormal visuomotor

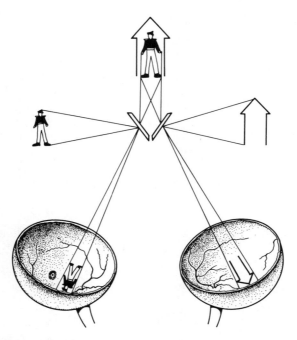

FIGURE 4.6. Abnormal localization or correspondence of images between the fixing eye and the deviated eye in strabismus.

behavior and the characteristics that any testable hypothesis about strabismus must explain.

As nature would have it though, there are, of course, persons in "inbetween" states who at times demonstrate all of the characteristics of the strabismic model described earlier and at other times appear to have perfectly straight eyes without any sensory anomalies. These have been termed intermittent deviations to signify that they are sometimes present and sometimes not. They rightly belong in the category of strabismus that we are discussing, and their behavior must be accounted for within any general theory. My reason for including them is that they possess the central attributes of the strabismic state: abnormal ocular posture, abnormal inhibition and localization in the central visual field of the deviated eye. I do not believe that strabismus, as defined earlier, represents only a difference in degree but not in kind from other states with which it is often lumped, such as phorias (latent visual axis deviations), or as simply another step along a continuum of oculomotor disorders. Rather, strabismus is a change of state that has almost nothing in common with "phorias." On the other hand, intermittent strabismus will furnish us, when carefully studied, important clues regarding the mildest anomalies of the central nervous system accounting for strabismus.

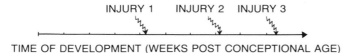

ERA OF STRABISMUS (RESPONSE TO INJURY)

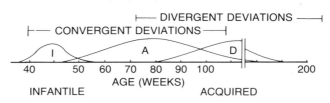

FIGURE 4.7. Distribution of the different types of strabismus seen at different times of development.

A Neurodevelopmental Theory of Strabismus

Let us now come to the theory itself. Strabismus is a specific response to an insult/injury of the central nervous system that, most importantly, occurred in a specific period (time) of development of the visual system and that may have both genetic and epigenetic components. It is the timing of the insult in development rather than the nature of the insult that gives rise to the discernible characteristics we identify with each clinical type of strabismus. The response to the injury comes from a very limited repertoire of responses that can occur within the visual system during that particular epoch of development. The clinical phenomenon of the response to injury may appear immediately but may be delayed until later (Figure 4.7). The reason for the delay in appearance is not apparent but may involve the maturation of components of the visual nervous system coupled with environmental factors that act as triggers to elicit the clinical symptomatology, that is, lessening hyperopia, reducing the accommodative demand for distance fixation combined with an increased interest in and need for distance fixation, may result in the onset of early intermittent divergent deviations in childhood.

The central nervous system's stereotyped response to injury resulting in strabismus consists of two components: loss of function(s) and adaptation to this loss. At this time, it is far from clear which of the behaviors of the strabismic patient's visuomotor system can be assigned to the former or the latter. If, however, the main tenets of the hypothesis, particularly its anatomical postulates, hold up on testing, it should be possible not only to make these assignments but also to predict other behaviors, such as the response to therapy. Let us, before we examine the anatomical details and the sequence in which I believe the events of the injury occur in strabismus, examine several corollaries of the basic hypothesis. First, the observed behaviors or characteristics of strabismus are the external manifestations of the dysmorphology of the central nervous system which is the result of the developmental injury. Second, careful study of the strabismic patient's behavior,

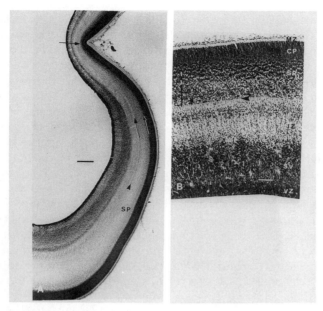

FIGURE 4.8. (A) Visual cortex of a 15-week-old fetus during formation of the subplate zone. Different stages can be seen along the curvature of the occipital cortex. At the depth of the calcarine fissure (arrow), there is a thin presubplate zone, while at the border of the calcarine cortex, formation of the second cortical plate is seen between the arrows. (B) Plastic 1 μm thick section of monkey visual cortex during the formation of the second cortical plate. MZ, marginal zone; SP_U, upper subplate; SP_L, lower subplate; IZ, intermediate zone; SV, subventricular; VZ, ventricular zone. From Kostovic I, Rakic P. Developmental history of the transient subplate zone in the visual and somatosensory cortex of the Macaque monkey and human brain. *J Comparative Neurology* 297:441–470, 1990. Copyright © 1990 Alan R. Liss. Reprinted by permission of Wiley-Liss, a division of John Wiley and Sons, Inc.

both sensory and motor, yields important insights into the nature and extent of the injury that produced the strabismus. It follows then that by studying and cataloging the abnormal behaviors of strabismus, we will be provided with an inverted telescope through which to examine the developing visual system to the point in time at which the event (the injury) occurred. Third, because of the very global nature of central nervous system development, careful study of the strabismic patient will yield evidence, though probably subtle, of defects in development of other systems, for example, auditory, somasthetic, motor, and early developmental learning, which, although mild, nevertheless accompany the developmental defect we recognize as strabismus. But more about that later (see Chapter 9).

Let us first choose an anatomical site where this injury might occur. I am led to choose the visual cortex as the most likely site of the injury that results in strabismus from such considerations as the time at which structures mature in the central nervous system, the lack of accompanying neurodevelopmental disease, the "plasticity" with which strabismus phenomenology adapts itself to changes wrought by growth and development of the infant and child, and the resistance of strabismus to a multiplicity of therapeutic interventions. To be more specific, I am postulating that the most likely candidate for the site of involvement is the area of the cortex immediately beneath the cortical plate, known as the subplate (Figure 4.8). As we have seen, it is a neurological structure that appears during ontogenesis of the nervous system, flourishes for a time, and then disappears when its function is completed, in accord with a mechanism consistent with the generation of strabismus. Let us summarize and review to this point what we have learned about the subplate. After their generation, neurons in the ventricular and subventricular zones of the neural tube subsequently migrate by glial guides to their final destinations in the developing central nervous system. Before invading the cortical plate of the central nervous system to form the layered structure of the fetal cortex (not the same structure as the adult cortex) they pass through the subplate immediately beneath the "cortex to be." This future cortex is bounded by a primitive cell-containing marginal zone comprising early-generated neurons defining the subpial layer of the cortex and a rich neuropil defining the subplate layer. The latter is far larger in extent than its cortical zone proper at this stage of development and contains, as we have seen, intracortical and thalamic afferents as well as its own population of neurons, which form synapses with each other and with geniculate afferents within the layer as well. These synapses are destined to disappear as is this neuronal population. This subplate layer rich in immunoreactive protein could well play a role in assigning destinations, connections, or both to the migrating cortical neurons destined for the mature cortex. This is the stage and the locus that contain all of the elements involved in proximity and connected by sets of synapses destined to disappear in normal circumstances.

It is the *interruption* of this normal pattern of behavior—emergence, flourishing development, and eventual death and disappearance—that results in the persistence of neural networks, which are not pruned back. This process is the core of the hypothesis I propose. It is during this phase of luxuriant synaptogenesis in the subplate layer when, as far as the visuomotor system is concerned, cells have not reached their final destination and "everything is connected to everything else" that atavistic sets of connections abound and are maintained. When these become operative later, they give rise to the sensory and motor behaviors we recognize as the essence of strabismus: abnormal ocular posture, evidence of an unusual type of suppression in the deviated eye, and abnormal topographical localization in this eye as well. Synaptogenesis, conceived of in this light, is a two-stage process, production and elimination, slightly offset in time (Figure 4.9). Production of synapses begins about the seventh month of pregnancy and reaches a peak at about birth. Starting slightly later, a process of "dying back" or interruption of synapses occurs that reduces the number (and probably type) of synapses, producing the biphasic curve typical of the process as a whole. Most probably, as well, the primitive neurons of this subplate zone are undergoing cell death, with that layer's gradual disappearance accompanying these latter events. This specific event, the *failure* of the "dying back" process, is the abnormal event leading to strabismus. Strabismus is, in its clinical phenomenology, the expression of the abnormal connectivity existing in the central nervous system. Primi-

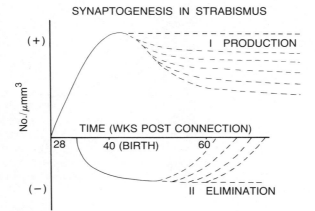

FIGURE 4.9. Process of synaptogenesis, which consists of two phases: synapse production and synapse elimination. In strabismus it is synapse elimination that is prematurely curtailed, leading to the survival of an excess of synapses.

tive synaptic connections, probably programmed during the wait in the subplate layer of the cortex and executed then or after the neurons arrive at their destination in the cortical layers, do not disappear and, as a result, abnormal connections persist within the cortex, a true dystrophy of connections.

Can we sharpen our question further: Where does this abnormality most likely occur? Although no firm answer to this question exists at present, we can direct our search to certain specific areas. As the macula is involved, its representation at every level of the visual cortex is suspect. And due to the anatomical peculiarities of its representation, the 17–18 border area, because it represents the vertical midline of the macula as well as the visual field as a whole, is a prime suspect (Figure 4.10). The abnormalities of the 17–18 border area found in albino animals suggests that this might be a place to look. A second anatomical site might well be the commissural fibers uniting the two halves of the visual field which normally carry only binocular connections from the 17–18 border area. In our model of strabismus, they would carry, in addition to these fibers, abnormal connections between the maculas and the peripheral visual fields (Figure 4.11). So the splenium of the corpus callosum is another anatomical area for potential study. What has been said earlier and illustrated diagrammatically would seem to suggest that the primary receptive cortex (area 17) and the peristriate cortex (area 18 particularly) are the only anatomical sites for these abnormal connections. This is not so. Rather, the abnormal connections could be present at any site in the visuomotor system where the visual fields, including the maculas, the vertical midline, and the peripheral visual fields, are represented. In fact, as is often the case in the central nervous system, a defect in neural tissue at one site gives rise to a cascade of defects downstream from the original locus. We present the anatomical aspects involving the striate and peristriate cortex because its anatomy is so familiar and well studied and because there is some suggestion in

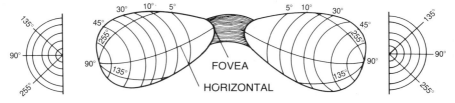

FIGURE 4.10. Normal binocular visual field and its anatomical representation in the calcarine cortex. Binocular connections between the two halves of the visual fields exist almost exclusively at the vertical midline strip of the field and are represented at the 17–18 border of the visual cortex and in the splenium of the corpus callosum. Adapted from Eye, Brain and Vision. By David H. Hubel. Copyright © 1988 by Scientific American Library. Reprinted with permission by W.H. Freeman and Company.

the animal literature that the 17–18 border area, the vertical meridian, and the callosal connections may be involved in animal models of strabismus. These models, however, are all generated on a basis conceptually very different than ours.

To summarize the essence of the model to this point, Figure 4.12 presents in stepwise fashion how the process unfolds.

Let us look again at the phenomenology of strabismus in the light of this conception and spell out some of its predictions. The abnormal cortical connections between the macular area of the fixing right eye in the illustration and the macula and nasal retina of the deviated left eye provide an anatomical basis for inhibition of the sensory input from this deviated eye. They also, at the same time, provide a basis for the existence of the abnormal localization phenomenon we call abnormal retinal correspondence. The peculiarities of suppression, its variability with the size of the test object, and its switching behavior between eyes as fixation shifts from eye to eye become comprehensible if one conceives of these connections in this fashion. According to the hypothesis, they are *reciprocal* connections, so information can flow in either direction (Figure 4.13). They provide a

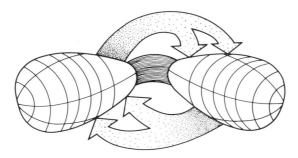

FIGURE 4.11. Abnormal connections between the macula of the fixing eye and the peripheral visual field (nasal retina) in convergent strabismus.

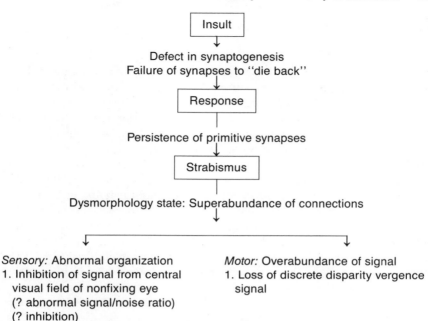

FIGURE 4.12. Steps in the development of strabismus.

network that can, at one and the same time, inhibit almost any incoming visual signal from either eye, yet provide information on its localization in space that will accurately reflect the receptors being stimulated in the retina. Both of these tasks are essential to adapting the visual world of the strabismic to permit the highest levels of function possible.

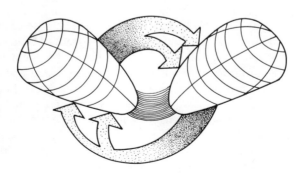

FIGURE 4.13. Bidirectional flow of information necessary to permit the rapid alternation of fixation between the two eyes and the abnormal localization characteristic of strabismus.

Equal Volumes of Disconnections Sweep Out Unequal Areas of Visual Field

There is a critical notion that must be assimilated here to make our theory comprehensible. It involves two facts embedded in the very structure of the cortex. The first is its very monotonous columnar arrangement. By observing its growth or microscopic anatomy one cannot tell whether cortex is processing visual information from the fovea or from the peripheral visual field (the machinery looks the same for both periphery and center). In contrast, the retina has a rich and variegated anatomy. The second is cortical magnification. Whereas 1 cubic millimeter of cortex processes $1°$ of visual information from the cortex representing the fovea, it may process $10°$ of visual information from the periphery. And that is the key in strabismus to the plasticity and areal extent of suppression and the localization of visual objects in space. One degree of connections at the macula of the fixing eye will be disconnected to $10°$ of peripheral retina and vice versa because of the persistence of connections going both ways! The volumes are the same. These atavistic connections should have been destroyed long ago but because they persist they give rise to the very unusual sensory phenomena in the central visual field of the deviated eye (and the fixing eye as well) in strabismics. The very rigidity of the cortical anatomy dictates the situation. The effect, when projected into the binocular visual field, is vastly different because of cortical magnification.

Finally, this abnormal array of binocular connections between the cortical representation of the macula area of the fixing eye and the extensive area of the peripheral, nonmacular retina of the nonfixing eye constitute the *abnormal disparity signal* to the vergence motor system. Instead of receiving a sharp, spatially localized, small-scale disparity signal to minutely adjust the ocular posture aligning the two foveas on the object of regard (Figure 4.14) (the role the fusional vergence system constantly plays in normal binocular vision), the vergence control system receives a veritable torrent of binocular signal between very disparate areas of the visual fields, resulting in the abnormal ocular posture we observe.

This anatomically grounded hypothesis permits us to think about strabismus and the variety of ways it presents clinically from several different viewpoints. First, the temporal aspect becomes more intelligible in terms of known principles of central nervous system development: The earlier in development the insult occurs, the more abnormal (in terms of connections) the response will be and the earlier the clinical condition is likely to present. This would constitute the group of patients we observe during infancy and whom we diagnose as having so-called congenital or infantile esotropia. Recognize that from the viewpoint I am proposing here, all strabismus is congenital or, really, prenatal and perinatal, as the developmental processes that give rise to it occur at that time. Birth is truly accidental because when it occurs, these processes are already underway and are destined to continue well into infancy.

The later the insult, the more normal the central anatomy will be and the later the onset of the recognizable clinical condition. It is more obvious that environ-

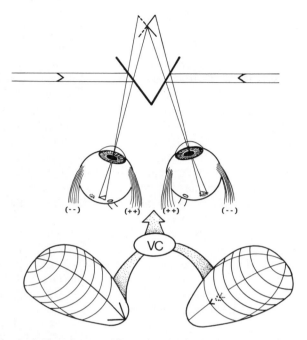

FIGURE 4.14. Motor consequence of the abnormal wiring of the visual cortex, which results in an abnormal disparity signal to the vergence control system. VC = Vergence Controller.

mental factors play a role in this form of strabismus. These examples of strabismus that we ordinarily call "acquired" are not, in fact, "acquired" at all. Rather, other factors come to play the role of precipitating agents (such as the development of hyperopia or the intensive use of the near-accommodative-convergence reflex by the infant) that trigger the onset of the clinical syndrome. But the anatomical groundwork in abnormal, superabundant connections has been laid down long before these events come to pass.

From this anatomical viewpoint the direction of the abnormal ocular posture becomes more intelligible. The earlier (both phylogenetically and ontogenetically) convergent system is vulnerable to injury early in development. The later (younger) divergent system is vulnerable to injury later in development. The direction the eyes assume then becomes an indicator of when in the developmental process of the visuomotor system the injury occurred, but is not in itself the etiology of the strabismus.

Let us reexamine the basic model of strabismus, admittedly a generalized and abstract one, from two viewpoints that now can be combined in our conception of strabismus. The two viewpoints to be combined are the anatomical constraints placed by the hypothesis: It has definite things to say about how the visuomotor system is miswired. The second is the observed phenomenology of strabismus, for example, the motor parameters of strabismus we observe clinically, such as a large size (and variability, if any) of the angular deviation. These might suggest, for example, the existence of broad and extensive abnormal connections between the two visual fields and perhaps an element of instability of the abnormal connections; the process is still going on—abnormal connections are being made and broken simultaneously—and has not reached a stable state. This may have, when its meaning is understood in terms of visuomotor development, important therapeutic consequences in the future. To take another example, the extent and nature of accompanying disturbances in oculomotor behavior—from the very minor, such as saccadization of pursuit, particularly pursuit away from the primary position (when unaccompanied by other visuomotor system defects), to more significant defects, such as monocular optokinetic nystagmus abnormalities and "upshoot" in adduction—become important not because they "cause" the strabismus (most certainly they do not) but because they, too, specify what other motor subsystems were under development at the time of the insult and perhaps provide us with clues to the nature of the defect necessary to produce the disturbances. I find it hard to believe that they are due to the absence or failure of development; rather, they represent the failure of primitive neural circuitry to be pruned back to a more efficient, smaller, more flexible and adapted normal circuitry. This question remains unanswered and will obviously be a subject of fruitful exploration by the clinician, the oculomotor physiologist, the model builder, and the psychophysicist working in cooperation with neural imagers. The important point is that these associated subsystem abnormalities are signposts; they tell us how the output side of the visuomotor system was being put together, probably many subsystems at once, when the basic insult occurred. Also important to note is that *time* is our guideline. When does the defect make its appearance? Was the basic deviation there some weeks or months before other behaviors manifested or did they occur together? Did one have to be changed in some way (therapeutic intervention) before the other became manifest? If so, why and how might this fit into an evolving model of strabismus? These questions were so puzzling and mysterious when we asked them previously that we were often tempted not to ask them at all; now, we have places in which to look for answers, which, even if complex, nevertheless seem to fit into a coherent framework of neurological development. This, in part known and in part still to be discovered, framework of neurological development of the visuomotor system is our matrix and our groundwork. Strabismus is our probe of its intricacies. Detailed knowledge of its anatomy and function is our goal.

Again, turning to our model of strabismus and combining the constraints of the hypothesis with the basic body of clinical and psychophysical observation, we are led to examine the sensory behavior of the strabismic from a new viewpoint. The lexicon of the strabismic sensory world is filled with such terms as suppression scotoma, facultative suppression, obligatory suppression, first-degree fusion, and unharmonious or harmonious correspondence. What do these terms mean? With respect to clarifying our understanding of disordered sensory processing, I believe that they tend to obscure rather than illuminate the phenomenon they are used to describe. Yet the central core of the hypothesis would predict that observed sensory behaviors examined in static (eyes still) or dynamic states (eyes moving in a saccadic, pursuit, vergence, or combined mode) should tell us a great deal about the nature, extent, type, and degree of disordered connections in the portion of the central visual field involved. For example, is position or motion processed within the central visual field of the deviated eye? Can this information, even if it is excluded from the conscious awareness of the subject, be utilized to originate and perform an accurate saccadic or pursuit eye movement? Although data on the psychophysics of the scotoma in strabismus are extant, more data need to be gathered. And the field should prove to be a fertile one, with a robust infrastructure of understanding coming from a convergence and complementarity of developmental, anatomical, neurophysiological, and psychophysical observation and experimentation. From the processing of color, contrast, spatial orientation, frequency, and the like, to motion detection and analysis, the information gained by the systematic study of their loss (rare) or distortion (common) within the central visual field of the deviated strabismic eye should help clarify our ideas of how and in what order they are processed binocularly for they are obviously processed quite normally under monocular viewing conditions in the strabismic patient. In my formulation thus far, I have implied that the loss of information in the central visual field of the deviated eye, as a result of these superabundant connections, must be taken to indicate an inhibition or editing out of signals present there. This is ingrained in the approach I have learned as a clinician and I have clung to it. However, it may well be that the phenomenon itself, suppression of information in the central visual field of the deviated eye, is not that at all; rather, the miswiring may result in an increased level of "noise," too much traffic in the circuits, that prevents the signal from being abstracted from this background (Figure 4.15). I believe the evidence indicates that all these premature, early-generated synapses are excitatory in nature. Careful analysis of the psychophysics of the central visual field of the deviated eye from the viewpoint of abnormal connections between the eyes should, however, help settle the question of the nature of the interaction. More about this later (see Chapter 7).

In still another area, abnormal localization of objects in space by the deviated eye, so-called abnormal correspondence, not only does the theory provide an obvious explanation but it also would not be tenable without such a phenomenon: The fovea of the fixing eye is, in fact, connected via functioning anatomical pathways to a whole series of points in the visual field of the deviated eye. This immediately accounts for the ubiquity of the observed phenomenon in strabismus (and its absence in any other form of oculomotor disturbance), and also accounts for some tantalizing aspects of its behavior, for example, its variability under different testing conditions. But that is only the beginning of the story, for changes in the output behavior of the eye muscles after surgery, in response to a given motor impulse, appear to change this correspondence. It is changed in ways that have not been systematically studied, though there is broad agreement that the

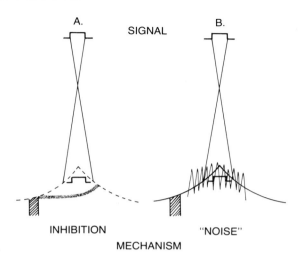

FIGURE 4.15. Inhibition in the central visual field of the deviated eye (A) versus the elevated "noise" level producing an abnormal "signal-to-noise" ratio (B).

correspondence shifts to preserve the localization state of the central visual field. Topologically, the fovea maintains connections with a vast array of points in the deviated eye. Depending on one's taste then, these arrays could be viewed as "abnormal" (the classical way) or "normal" (the anatomical way). I prefer the latter. Yet, the model suggests that this type of feedback behavior (a mismatch between innervational input and muscle output), of which normal persons are ordinarily unaware in binocular vision, is a commonplace and predictable pattern in strabismus. The goal of the pattern is to maintain objects imaged in the central visual fields of both eyes as close to location in the same place in space as possible. Understanding how this might occur under static and dynamic conditions in strabismus may tell us a great deal about how normal persons process, integrate, and differentiate position and motion signals originating from eye or image movements. The process is "opened up," so to speak, by the miswiring of the strabismus. And it is not uniform over the entire visual field. Some areas of the field are apparently normal in their connections (correspondence); others are not. Changes in correspondence (localization) in some cases are slow to adapt and lag behind the motor behavior. Why? What sequence do they follow in adapting? At what level do they adapt? Is the adaptation the same in a moving visual environment (OKN or VOR stimulation) as in a stationary environment? What model of miswiring would produce a mislocalization insensitive to stimulation close to the brain stem output (vestibular stimulation) but responsive to gaze stimulation (up versus down gaze)? These and many other questions await the imagination and efforts of clinicians and research workers anxious to "fill in the blanks" for the normal person as well as the strabismic. And from the viewpoint expressed in the central premise of the hypothesis, that anatomical miswiring accounts for observed defects, it should be possible to do so.

Let us now turn our attention to potential defects in the hypothesis. In simplest terms, the hypothesis states that what we observe from the outside is a replica of what is inside, that is, we are observing end-organ sensorimotor behavior that, if we knew the connections and the code, will tell us exactly where and how the visuomotor brain is miswired. Further, the hypothesis states that if we look carefully enough at the phenomena we are observing, they will likely tell us where, when, how, and perhaps why the miswiring occurred. With a hypothesis so sweeping, the first possibility to be considered is that it is dead wrong. Assuming that it is so, in proving it totally wrong we will gather important data on our patients (see Chapters 7 and 8), on their strabismus phenomenology (see Chapter 6), on their visuomotor nervous system development (Chapters 2 and 10), on its anatomy (Chapter 11). The picture that emerges, although not corresponding to the hypothesis, will, in itself, furnish a beginning for the generation of other hypotheses conforming more closely to the newly gathered data. In point of fact, the effort expended in disproving any hypothesis more than rewards those who prove it false. I have no pretense that my hypothesis is anything more than a very simple attempt to bring into congruence the body of knowledge that has emerged in the seventh through ninth decades of this century on the formation and function of the early nervous system with the growing body of knowledge about the variety of timing of insults to that developing system with the clinical phenomenology of strabismus. I consider the latter an example of a specific dysmorphology of a particular, important epoch of that development, synaptogenesis. If, in fact, strabismus has nothing whatsoever to do with synaptogenesis, we will have learned a great deal about the process in humans that we did not know before. My intuition then is that the information which becomes available will tell us where to look further.

A second possibility is that the hypothesis, though not dead wrong, is however flawed, in that it focuses on the wrong part of the system. My reasons for choosing a site so high in the visual nervous system (namely, cortex, primary receptive and early associative) is that so much is preserved and normal in strabismus. Let us not forget that the neuraxis matures phylogenetically. The more primitive is ready before the more elaborate. Strabismus does not affect the lower motor neurons, nor does it seem to me to affect supranuclear gaze mechanisms, except in special cases and then only as an associated, not primary, defect. Strabismus is, above all else, a disorder of the most elaborate processing of binocular, not monocular, information and that is where we should look for clues to its nature. Though I have described it in a very specific manner and placed its disordered anatomy in a very specific region—the primary receptive visual cortex, area 17, visual associative cortex, area 18, and their commissural connections—it need not be there at all. Rather, its site may in fact be located in any of a number of areas in the visuomotor system where commissura exist, where functional halves of the visual field are put together binocularly and where a specific oculomotor behavior is programmed—disjunctive eye movements to center the object of regard on both the foveas. If this is accomplished, for example, in the right peristriate cortex, much as language is processed in the left cortex, then this is where we should look to find the specific anatomical defects that the hypothesis predicts and we should look at the vertical midline of the visual field, where those defects are likely to begin. The reader can reflect on how much more elaborate our knowledge of the visuomotor system will be if we find that area, explore it with various probes, and determine that it appears normal in strabismus. The search will then be narrowed even further!

Let us consider the case that strabismus is "functional," that is has no specific anatomic grounding. In many ways, this is our current conception of the entity and we even talk in some of its classification systems in terms that suggest the conception, for example, "excesses" of convergence or divergence, "insufficiencies" of the same, and "basic" or "pseudodivergence" type of deviation. These words imply functions or defects in functions about which we know little. They are, however, from my viewpoint, not doors with thresholds through which we can walk but walls that box in our thinking. Until we fully understand what convergence is, it is unlikely that we will come to a meta-understanding of what its "excess" is. And function, whatever it be, must have a grounding in structure. It vivifies structure without doubt but it must have a physically realizable network through which it operates to produce its ends. If, in fact, the defect in strabismus is at this most abstract level, a functional one, we must still find a site or sites in the visual nervous system at which that abstraction becomes concrete and a network of neurons behave in a pattern that produces strabismus.

As a final point, could strabismus be a disorder of an end organ, the eye (or retina) and/or extraocular muscles? Although this concept has a hallowed pedigree in the pantheon of ophthalmology, and is associated with names like von Graefé and Scobee, it is, or so it seems to me, putting the chicken coop before either the egg or the chicken. I do not in any sense mean to belittle the concepts of others but if, in fact, such were the case, then for example, many skilled clinicians observing the retina in the eyes of strabismics or adjusting muscle tension in treating it have failed, in well over a century of conscious effort, to find even a subtle defect in the former or a cure of the condition in the latter. I fear the search must continue.

5
How Might We Classify Strabismus?

Man is the measure of all things.

Protagoras

A classification in medicine might be likened to a blueprint for construction of a house. The blueprint is not a very pretty or exciting work of art, but without it, there would be no house. A classification is, as we know from many areas in medicine, a singular activity, which when carried out on the deepest level of our understanding of diseases and their effects on the human organism, provides a scaffold (a blueprint of the mind, so to speak) on which entire generations of clinical and basic research efforts, of therapeutic trials, and of natural history studies of disease may be founded. At its best, a classification has many intellectual offspring that use it to test, to measure, and to guide, those efforts. The best classification systems have two properties that are embedded in their structure and endear them to all who use them. The first is a simple, unambiguous, easily grasped central principle to which all data (laboratory, clinical, historical, physical, and so on) may be related, for example, cardiac function in the American Heart Association Classification of heart disease. The second is a structure that does not necessitate the total storage capacity of our short-term memory. One need not carry a heavy tome to have access to and to utilize the classification. These two qualities are reciprocally related. The deeper and more penetrating our understanding of the entity we wish to classify, the simpler and more unambiguous will be the classification's central principle. From this arises a basic unity that enables us to perceive, in what may be a rich diversity of appearances, a common nature, combining many diverse phenomena within a manageable structure.

Although each of the current classifications of strabismus looks at the problem along one dimension (Figure 5.1), none penetrates deeply enough into the essence of the subject to encompass it. This is not said to disparage these classifications, but simply to point out that none of them fulfills even the first of the requisites—a unifying central principle around which all observations can be gathered. Neither "fusion," nor age of appearance, nor accommodative state, nor excesses and insufficiencies of vergences serve such a function. We do not know what "fusion" is, nor what its absence or presence may mean, nor what makes

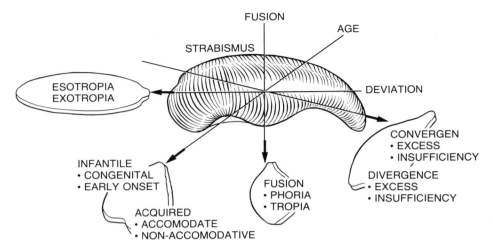

FIGURE 5.1. Each of the current classifications of strabismus views it from a unique standpoint, accounting for some but not all of its behaviors along a scalar dimension.

strabismus that appears conatally (rare) different from strabismus that presents perinatally (Days 0 to 28) or during the infantile period (1 to 12 months). Nor do we know why uncorrected hyperopia is associated with the onset of "acquired" (whatever that term means) esotropia in some, but not all by any means, childhood hyperopes. Each classification concentrates on a different dimension of the problem and, hence, classifies some but not all cases of strabismus. Each classification has its defects and perhaps nowhere is this more apparent than in clinical studies that use one or the other classification system. We may have reservations about any study purporting to detail the effects of spectacle treatment of accommodative esotropia if, for example, we are not provided with some notion of the age at which the process (strabismus) began and the residuum of normal binocular function the patient possessed when he or she became esotropic. The study may be as prospective, well designed, painstaking, detailed, and accurate as possible. Yet, without that critical variable, which is intrinsic to the nature of strabismus (and therefore must be built into any classification system), clinical studies purporting to show this or that effect will be suspect. As I have said in other contexts, a classification system is to (the nosology of) a disease as grammar, syntax, and basic vocabulary are to language. We are not yet, in strabismus, much above the level of infant babble. One has but to look at the progress that has been made in diabetic retinopathy, age-related macula degeneration, and retinopathy of prematurity to be aware of how far we have to go. For all these diseases, the story began with a classification system developed around a powerful idea understood by all and encompassing the clinical phenomenology that lent coherence to the clinical and basic studies. It should, on the other hand, be quite obvious to the reader how much easier these were to classify, as their fundamental pathology, much of their prepathological state, and a great deal of basic science directly concerned with the disease entities were well known prior to the generation of the classification. Furthermore, their pathology could be directly observed and their pathogenesis inferred from material at hand. Such is quite clearly not the case in strabismus today.

Having made at great length this prologue to the question of classification in strabismus, let me now state that I do not have one to give the reader. We are still in the early stage of development of our knowledge about strabismus though the condition has been around for millennia. The reason is that its matrix—the development of the visual nervous system—has only, within the last century, begun to emerge from the shadows. Within the last two to three decades, a clear-cut picture of the development of neural processing circuitry from the birth of neurons to transmitter pharmacology has emerged and we can begin to infer how vision might work at the level of the retina, lateral geniculate nucleus, and, in a very primitive sense, the primary and association visual cortices out to the level of oculomotor output. Yet this is the infrastructure that must underlie any comprehensive classification of strabismus worth its clinical name. These are the dimensions of the problem we face. That does not mean we cannot perform a useful thought experiment involving the principles that must be embedded in the classification of strabismus yet to come. Let us do that and see where the endeavor leads us.

1. First, we must, I believe, firmly embed strabismus in the matrix in which it belongs—an anomaly of neurodevelopment. I have, along these lines, postulated a *specific era*, synaptogenesis; a *specific process*, failure of synapses to "die back"; and an *anatomical site*, subplate of the cortex, in previous chapters as being the neural substrate responsible for strabismus clinical phenomenology in the generic model (Figure 5.2).
2. Let us assume for the moment that these three postulates are correct (highly unlikely!). Where do we go now? It is essential to break down the postulates into a classification that is usable, that is, to break down the *large and general eras* into more specific suberas, when the *specific process* is disturbed to give rise to a number of clinical states. Clearly, frustration of the process throughout synaptogenesis leads to an entirely different set of dysconnections (both in number and in type) than would be obtained if the process is disturbed only at its inception or termination. Remember how *time specific* injury is in the central nervous system (Figure 5.3). I would submit that any classification encompassing these ideas in this setting would have to account for (specify) at least two variables: (1) what has developed normally up to the insult (for that will be preserved); (2) what failed to develop both at the time of the insult and downstream from it, as so much of central nervous system development is cascade-like in its effect; that is, a small defect or change in conditions at one point in time can have many later effects on processes far removed in time and space from the initial defect.

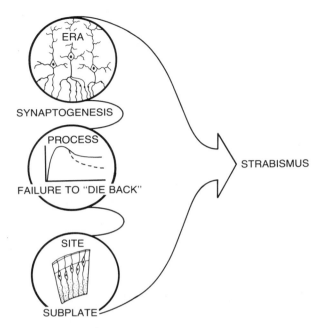

FIGURE 5.2. A classification system of strabismus should encompass a time, a process, and an anatomical site to account for the clinical phenomenology.

3. Any classification worth its clinical name should, as well, specify function; that is the name of the game in vision: what is preserved and intact, what is lost and likely never to develop further, and what is, by dint of our therapeutic manipulations (current or yet to be imagined), possible or likely to be recoverable. It is this last "gray zone" to which all or most of our intellect, talent, heart — disguised as our "therapeutic efforts"— should be devoted. The central nervous system, with its store of established functions, will get along quite nicely without us. We should waste no time or effort on what we cannot change and our classification should lead us to easily distinguish between these two and focus on the middle ground, which is our rightful sphere of influence.

What emerges from a set of considerations such as the preceding is, first, the idea that strabismus is not a curiosity occupying the time and effort of some bizarre group of like-minded clinicians without reference to any other body of medical knowledge, but rather, an example having much in common with other central nervous system developmental anomalies and, because of its open and studiable phenomenology, telling us a great deal about how the central nervous system is put together. Second, because of the varying clinical picture of strabismus, the accurate specification of its *site*, *time*, and *process* will yield manifold dividends as to what does what and when it takes place in the central

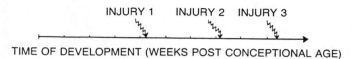

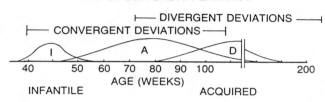

FIGURE 5.3. Time-specific injuries to the developing visuomotor vergence system result in anomalous behavior accounting for infantile esotropia (I), acquired esotropia (A), and exotropia (D). The clinical phenomenology reflects the time and the site of the injury.

nervous system. Third, investigation of how strabismus can be manipulated by interventions on our part (what can be improved) will give us insights into many areas of modifiability (plasticity) of the central nervous system function, in general, now closed to our imaginations.

In this chapter, I have not given the reader a classification "from on high." I have none. But I hope the reader grasps the immensity and yet the dimensions and limits of the task. In so doing, a first small step in completing it has been taken. Let me close by paraphrasing Protagoras' statement with which I opened this chapter. In strabismus, the developing brain is the measure of all things.

6
How Can We Look Anew at Strabismus?

If the doors of perception were cleansed, everything would appear to man as it is, infinite.
For man has closed himself up, til he sees all things through narrow chinks of his cavern.

William Blake

There is no more refreshing experience in medicine, and perhaps in all of science, than to look with fresh eyes at phenomena that have long since ceased to mystify us and to which we have become apathetic because we failed to understand their meaning. The mind "adapts" to what is mysterious in nature and in so doing trivializes it. Not because the phenomenon itself is trivial, but because our mind repeatedly fails to comprehend it and it therefore becomes an irritant around which we build an eschar to wall it off from our conscious thought processes. When, on the other hand, an explanation that suggests a rational basis for understanding arises, it is with a sense of joy and challenge that we look again at the once mysterious, then irritating, then trivial phenomenon. Let us do this with the phenomenology of strabismus in the clinic and examine the ways in which the new conception may enlighten us.

We begin, for didactic reasons only, by separating sensory and motor, not because there is any real separation between them—we see with our whole visuomotor brain. Rather, the duality of the system is enforced by our primitive conceptions of how the system works. It is much like the wave-particle duality of the photon of light or the electron; both viewpoints must be kept in consciousness to fully understand the behavior of the entity, though one aspect of its behavior may best be explained by employing one or the other frame of reference. So it is with strabismic dysmorphology: Its behavior is best accounted for clinically by examining it from the universal viewpoint of an excess or surplus of connections that we postulate are excitatory and reciprocal in nature, which means that a type of instant reversibility exists between the dysconnected areas. As a consequence, effects, although more subtle, from the nonfixing to the fixing eye can be expected as well as the reverse.

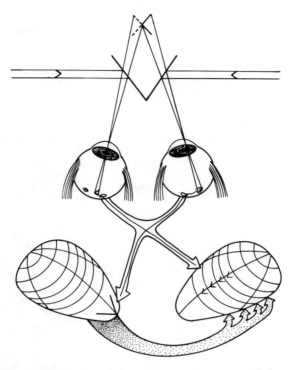

FIGURE 6.1. Abnormal connections existing between the macula and multiple sites in the peripheral visual field of the deviated eye in strabismus.

Motor Phenomenology

Now we look for some specific clinical consequences of this dysmorphology. Let us look first at the motor side of strabismus phenomenology, not because it is more important than the sensory side, but because it is the one most early and easily observed. Let us apply, in stepwise fashion, what our conception of the dysconnected innervational field might produce at various intervals of behavioral adaptation to the abnormal visuomotor state. In the earliest stages of strabismus, *after* it is present and the dysconnected synapses are operative, the first behavior that the observer should notice is an unstable or metastable state. Several networks may be operating at once (Figure 6.1), each seeking to achieve the best (highest) information state (capture the most cortical processing units available). This behavior may at times be extremely transient as one or another strategy (circuit) comes to be the one that maximizes the useful binocular "signal" (information from the two eyes) and minimizes the "noise" (interfering signal from the deviated eye) and, hence, is the one adopted. This period may, in fact, be so

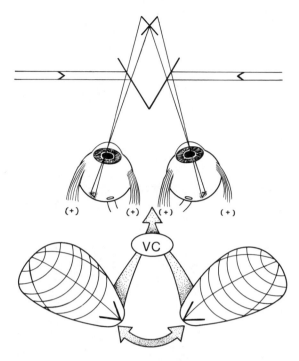

FIGURE 6.2. Stimulation of the macula of the deviated eye in strabismus. VC = Vergence Controller.

short as to escape our notice. But in those cases in which the phenomenon is observable, the concept we have evolved should predict certain motor behaviors. First, increasing the stimulus (its size, luminance, contrast, color saturation, motion, and so on) in the deviated eye should produce two sets of effects depending on (within limits) where the stimulus is placed. When placed into the peripheral visual field aligned with the macula of the fixing eye, the stimulus should produce an increase in the abnormal vergence signal and an increase in the deviation. Within limits, again probably set by the volume of dysconnected cortex rather than the mechanical limits of the dysjugate behavior, this process of increased vergence signal in response to increase–stimulus should continue to result in an increase in the angle of deviation. Conversely, stimulation of the macular region of the deviated eye should produce a decrease in the angle of deviation (again within limits superimposed by the residual excess of dysjugate signal coming from the peripheral area of the deviated eye) (Figure 6.2). We should then be able to observe in the early metastable state two specific types of motor behavior, each programmed by its connections, in opposite directions: one tending to increase dysjugacy, the other tending to reduce it. The consequences for potential therapy should be obvious.

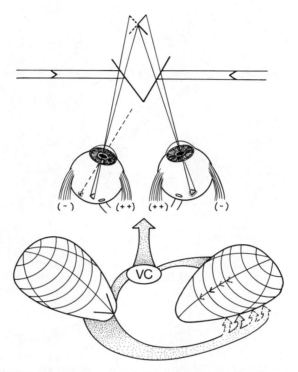

FIGURE 6.3. Adoption by the strabismic of a single set of visuomotor connections that account for the stabilization of the angle of strabismus. This is a developmental effect. VC = Vergence Controller.

It is unlikely that this behavior will persist, however, when the next stage of development of the motor behavior of strabismus unfolds. For here, the system has become adapted or in a sense "hardwired." Though I detest jargon, "hardwired" here as a purely descriptive term suffices when it means only that a metastable or unstable behavior has been abandoned and a particular set of connections adopted that stabilizes the abnormal signal and hence the abnormal ocular position (Figure 6.3). At that point, the motor behavior can be influenced from the peripheral visual field only, stimulation of the macula area of the deviated eye having lost the ability. Note here, as we examine the motor behavior of the strabismic, the heavy emphasis placed on the sensorimotor interaction. In my view one never exists without the other.

Still another motor phenomenon that may be easily observed is the "fixing" eye or the "field of fixation" of the two eyes. As we noted in Chapter 4, we are limiting ourselves in discussing this condition to the "generic model" of strabismus: equal visual acuity, no amblyopia. The angle of deviation, its magnitude, and its direction are not of concern to us except as they specify "fields" of abnormal

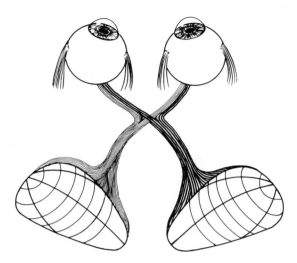

FIGURE 6.4. Representation of ocular dominance on an anatomical basis: capture of the most processing units in a given hemisphere by its visual input (the right hemisphere in this case).

connections and, more fundamentally, the stage in development when the insult occurred. We are aware at once of several things. First, the fixation behavior of the two eyes is almost never divided temporally 50/50 but rather 80/20, 70/30, or some such ratio. Second, we note that patterns of fixation switch occur at differing gaze angles in these patients. What do these phenomena mean? The former is, in the conception of strabismus that dominates this book, a manifestation of the "dominant eye" phenomenon referred to earlier. It represents the hemisphere that has the most processing units captured by its visual input (Figure 6.4). If it is the right hemisphere, the right eye will be dominant, and if it is the left hemisphere, the left eye will be dominant. After careful study I believe that eye dominance will be shown to have exactly the same distribution in strabismic and normal populations. Although standard teaching would suggest that in alternating strabismus, the alternating ratio or alternate usage of the two eyes should be equal, or nearly equal, we realize clinically that this is not often the case. The reason usually advanced for fixing this ratio of alternate usage is to maintain the acuity of both eyes nearly equal. I would point out that true and complete alternation is almost never observed in a strabismic patient. In spite of the fact that the visual acuity can be equal or nearly equal and there is no evidence of amblyopia. Furthermore, there may be subtle (and interesting) shifts of motor behavior—a distribution of fixation behaviors (Figure 6.5) between near and distant fixation, and oblique gazes with which all clinicians are familiar. Under our conception of strabismus, they do not have anything to do with the acuity of the eye (except in the limiting case where amblyopia has developed), but rather represent the visuomotor state that brings

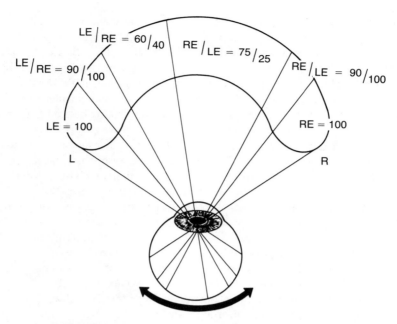

FIGURE 6.5. Parcellation of fixation behaviors between the two eyes in an alternating strabismic at a given fixation distance. LE = left eye, RE = right eye.

the *least* "noise" into the system. By "noise" here we understand that the strabismic brain has many patterns of innervation to choose from because of the dysconnectivity of the visuomotor system. In each field of gaze, then, that brain utilizes one of the patterns that permits (1) the most nearly "normal" sensory input (least inhibition of the deviated eye's stimulus and localization information) similar to the information in the macular area of the fixing eye, and (2) the least "abnormal" motor posture (tendency to reduce the angle of deviation toward zero). As long as similar images with similar information content and localization are available to the two eyes, however disparate their ocular position, these behaviors will be manifest. The reason for this is the coexistence of both normal connections and dysconnections in the strabismic visuomotor system. The coexisting normal connections drive the visuomotor system to (1) obtain maximum information from both eyes of the visual scene and (2) reduce to a minimum the deviation error and the correspondence error between the two eyes. These behaviors are coupled. It is, I believe, intrinsic behavior in the central nervous system to do such, and where the eyes are and what they are seeing at any given position in the field of gaze illustrate this principle.

What would this conception mean practically? First, alternation of fixation behaviors tells us these are fields where either right or left eye dominance comes closest to a normal innervation "set" (sensory and motor behavior most closely approaching normal) for the two eyes. Second, we should be able to demonstrate, by suitable, nondisruptive testing, differences in the motor and sensory phenomenology between eyes in a given field of gaze. For example, in gaze to the right, let us say that the right eye is exclusively used for fixation. Then, in right gaze we should by suitable (nondisruptive) testing be able to demonstrate a "smaller" scotoma (areal dimensions and depth) under binocular conditions in the deviated left eye, and a localization angle and deviation angle that are both smaller than with left eye fixation. Note that I stress that "nondisruptive" testing be used to demonstrate the phenomenon, for example, use of the space haploscope of Guyton, which maintains identical central and peripheral visual fields while making simultaneous sensory and motor measurements. This is critical, because the so-called "objective" methods of measurement (prisms, cover tests, red/green glasses, and so on) either disturb the visuomotor system and force it out of its natural state (cover tests) or transmit information from another adapted state (red/green or polaroid glasses) with a different innervational (sensory and motor) set.

To return to our topic, the exploration of what "alternation" means in the strabismic state, the theory would predict, first, the adoption of a strategy to minimize the sensory and motor innervation set over all possible ranges (dynamic) and positions (static) of gaze. Second, it would predict that one of the two eyes would be dominant in most, but not all fields of gaze and would remain so unless environmental conditions brought about a change in either input or output (for example, patches, surgery) or both, necessitating the adoption of another set of connections. It would predict that the "dominant" eye would, in fact, occur with about the same frequency as "eye dominance" occurs in the normal population. I believe the same phenomenon operates in the patient with alternating strabismus; that is, either the right or left hemisphere is dominant and the ipsilateral eye drives both eyes in the majority of fields of gaze. The behavior in the alternating strabismic, however, is not as absolutely proscribed as it is in the normal person and the other cortex (eye) can become dominant under some sensorimotor conditions. In fact, this type of behavior should be expected to occur and could easily be recorded on a clinical motility chart.

On a more subtle level, but one that is nevertheless discernible, the abnormal ocular posture (angle of deviation and dynamics of the movement itself) should change whenever the "nondominant" eye is forced (by nondisruptive methods) to fix in a field of gaze or make an eye movement to a field of gaze as the fixing eye of the pair. Several phenomena should occur. First, the abnormal ocular posture (angle of deviation) should change in the direction of increase rather than decrease (increase in "noise" → vergence signal increase → increased angle). Second, the scotoma mapped in the central visual field of the nonfixing ("forced" nondominant) eye should be larger than when measured under ordinary dominant eye testing conditions. And third, the abnormal localization in the central visual field in the nonfixing ("forced" nondominant) eye should deviate away from the adapted state. These should not be perfect mirror images of one another. It is not clear in which direction this change of localization should occur. My intuition suggests that it might be toward an increase in localization error. But it

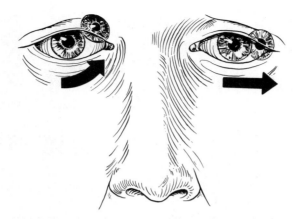

FIGURE 6.6. Loss of fixation by the dominant eye in the adduct position in "so-called inferior oblique overaction."

is something that can be clinically determined and is, I believe, specified by the dysconnection set or field for this eye (reciprocal connections).

Clinicians reading the preceding paragraphs may immediately object to the formulation presented on several grounds. The first of these is obvious. Children with strabismic eyes who have, for example, "overaction" of the inferior oblique will almost always fix the opposite eye in the field of gaze of the "overacting" inferior oblique. Fixation then becomes automatic between the adducting and abducting eye during the course of the gaze movement. This behavior is quite true and quite specific. But it has, I suggest, a completely different meaning. Here the macular area of, let us say, the dominant right eye is physically prevented by the abnormal vertical eye movement (innervation) from maintaining fixation (dominance) in the adducted field of gaze to the left. As the dominant right eye adducts and the vertical movement begins, this dominant eye loses fixation and the nondominant eye assumes fixation during this gaze movement and when the field of gaze is attained (Figure 6.6). The physical position of the eyes in the orbit during the movement and when its goal is attained intervenes to prevent the ordinary principles governing eye dominance from operating in this case. Parenthetically, it would be interesting to study whether therapy (surgery on the "overacting" oblique) influences this pattern. I would doubt that it does, but I base this doubt on my speculation as to the true nature of the apparent inferior oblique "overaction," which for me it is, most assuredly, not. This is, however, not germane to our subject.

Still another oculomotor behavior seemingly in contradiction to what the theory would predict is that of dissociated vertical deviation or divergence (DVD). Here, in a number of varied circumstances, an oculomotor behavior associated commonly with strabismus changes the fixation pattern in otherwise alternating

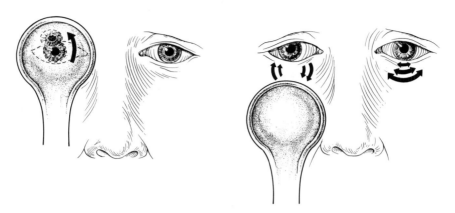

FIGURE 6.7. "Scale balance" or "rocking" behavior observed in both eyes after removal of the cover from one eye in DVD.

strabismus. How can this be? And how is this behavior explained within the framework of the dysconnection hypothesis? First, let us examine in some detail how the behavior is evoked. Well known is the use of a darkening wedge placed before the fixing eye (Bielschowsky phenomenon) to produce a downward movement in the dissociated (elevated) eye. In fact, any nonspecific stimulation of the macular area of the dominant, fixing eye will elicit a similar movement in the dissociated eye—a bright light (glare source?), a prism, a cover placed swiftly in front of the fixing eye and quickly withdrawn, and even at times a very light red glass will be enough to bring about a shift in fixation behavior. Still another way to provoke the deviation is to neutralize the horizontal deviation with prisms (or surgery) so that the object of regard is close to, if not, bimacular. Again, the abnormal behavior manifests itself.

It is not our purpose here to describe in detail the clinical phenomenology of DVD. This is done very well elsewhere in great detail. Several other phenomena are worthy of mention. The first of these is the "scale balance" phenomenon often observed in the presence of DVD (Figure 6.7). By this I mean the "settling down" of the size of the vertical deviation as the patient becomes binocular again after, for example, prism cover measurements (by right eye and left eye fixation) of the size of the vertical deviation in the opposite eye. The second is the rotary movement observed in the fixing eye when the deviating eye is covered and drifting upward and outward to its resting position. Although not apparently conjugate, the fixing (dominant) eye is nevertheless receiving an innervational signal as evidenced by the movement. Still a third sensory phenomenon is the presence of significant (measurable) vertical scotomata in these nonfixing, deviated eyes, but the absence, in most cases, of any evidence of bimacular sensation, even when tested for with disparate targets. Finally, although not strictly limited to such patients, DVD occurs most frequently and commonly with infantile esotropia

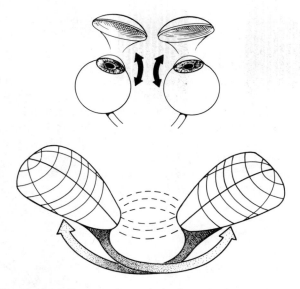

FIGURE 6.8. Hypothesized disconnections existing between the macular regions of the two eyes in DVD.

and is accompanied by congenital nystagmus. These indicate a very early insult to the developing visuomotor system.

How then do we relate this disparate and unusual clinical phenomenology as presented by DVD within the framework of our alternating strabismic patient? The explanation, I believe, lies in the specific type of dysconnection that occurs in DVD. In fact, DVD gives us the best current example of a dysconnection state of a peculiar and localized type. The clinical phenomenology of DVD is best explained by a total dysconnection between the macular regions of the two eyes (Figure 6.8). In contrast to other clinical examples of strabismus in which both maculas remain connected and normally coexist with abnormal peripheral connections, in the presence of DVD, I postulate that no normal bimacular connections exist. It is the consequence of a very early developmental error. In other words, what we observe clinically is that any change that diminishes the stimulus information (weight) in the fixing macula (the darkening wedge, the slit lamp beam) will cause the dominance of this macula to begin to shift to the nonfixing macula. A programmed series of eye movements will then occur in which the nonfixing macula descends to the horizontal plane to assume ocular dominance. The other macula simultaneously assumes the vertically deviated position. The essence of the phenomenon is the complete *absence* of binocular connections between the two maculas. Why vertical? Because of the complete absence of binocular connections and, hence, the complete absence of the development of horizontal macula vergence reflex mechanisms that depend on the connections for their establishment, we have persisting, instead, a mesencephalic control system much like the systems described by Nashold and Seaber and Jampel and Fells, discovered during surgical ablations to control movement disorders in the former and lesions of the mesencephalon in the latter.

The pathways for this vertical eye movement are, of course, presently unspecified and remain to be elucidated. That they are associated with this most striking utromacular abnormality is at least a clue to their starting point.

Both of these visuomotor patterns, inferior oblique "overaction" and DVD, are not counterarguments to the theory but rather special cases with patterns of visuomotor behavior that call for explanations beyond the limits of our current understanding of the dysconnections resulting in the clinical phenomenology of strabismus.

Sensory Phenomenology

The previous section, although devoted to describing principally specific motor patterns of behavior, nevertheless treated, in passing, the sensory side as well. These two sides cannot be conceptually disentangled. Here we devote our attention to the sensory phenomenology as an expression of the dysconnection. In the visual world our maculas are "captured" momentarily by an object of regard, which we inspect for an instant before sliding the maculas beneath the next object that captures our attention and interest. It is all done effortlessly (Figure 6.9). We adjust our ocular posture to maintain the world centered on our maculas by employing at least five motor subsystems: saccadic, pursuit, vergence, vestibular, and fixation. All are well integrated and all work to convey a more or less accurate perception of the external world seen as a single percept and in depth. Let us begin by examining the sensation of the strabismic in much the same way. If it were possible to somehow tap into the conscious visual perception of the strabismic, how would it differ from ours? Remarkably little, I believe. It is a visual world, again, macula centered. Motor subsystems at the instantaneous beck and call of that macula respond by bringing visual objects of interest effortlessly onto the macula. In our model of alternating strabismus, the macula of either eye can be employed to inspect the image and a shift between the eyes is accomplished leaving no conscious trace for the most part. It all looks very much as our world with "things in their place" does. How does this come about? The answer, I submit, arises out of the very nature of these abnormal connections. They permit two effects to occur simultaneously: a flexible, in time and space, "blanking" of the central visual field of the deviated eye and a topographical realignment of the spatial values of that central visual field to agree with the topography of the spatial values of the central visual field of the dominant macula. Let us now look at some of the qualities these connections must possess if they are to achieve the stable visual world for the strabismic so like our own. To do so, these connections must exist in abundance, as I believe they do. They must be able to be reciprocally employed, that is, to carry messages both ways, and

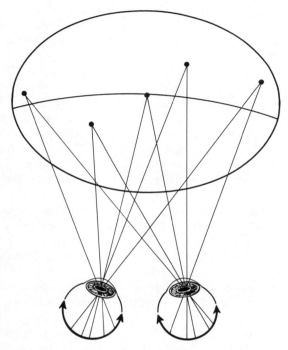

FIGURE 6.9. Shifts of gaze involving saccadic pursuit and vergence changes as well as vestibular and fixation subsystems that main stability in the visual world.

therefore should exist in parallel. They must be of the "point-to-field" type to accommodate this condition, i.e. one degree of macula cortical representation being equivalent to ten or fifteen degrees of peripheral cortical representation. And they must subserve a sensory function—to inhibit only that information from the central visual field of the deviated eye (including both macula and periphery) that might conceivably be confused with information conveyed to consciousness by the central visual field of the fixing eye while permitting all other useful information to pass unchallenged—and a spatial mapping function—to restore to normal or near-normal topography the central visual field of the deviated eye by remapping the spatial values to conform to those of the central visual field of the fixing eye. It should be noted that this plays no role in producing a fusion response (except in very particular cases). Rather, for the purpose of generating motor system commands, it brings the two spatial maps into register; finally the connections themselves signal the vergence control center which determines the error in ocular alignment (the angle of deviation and its sign). The first two are our concern here. What behaviors would such a set of dysconnections imply? First, because of their "point-to-field" representation between macula and periphery, they give rise to the following effects: The larger the target occupying the macula and near periphery of the fixing eye, the larger the area of suppression of a similar target in the deviated eye. The targets that best bring this out are targets with identical contours. It is these that produce the phenomenon. Targets with dissimilar contours do not ordinarily produce this phenomenon; when they do, it is not as marked on testing as it is for identical contours. The key is that by enlarging the target extent in the macula or near periphery of the central visual field of the fixing eye, the area of inhibition (connections stimulated) in the central visual field of the deviated eye increases. This effect has limits in that if the target is made large enough it can extend beyond the area of dysconnection and be imaged by both eyes. The limits of these effects are unknown at present and constitute a broad and important area of necessary and new study. They might very well be as accurate a definition of the dysconnected areas as any we have on hand clinically.

Still another effect is the "surround-center" interaction. Peripheral contours presented in the central visual field of the fixing eye have the effect of suppressing more intensely the macular region of the deviated eye (Figure 6.10). Once again the effect has anatomical limits beyond which it breaks down. These are not known with any certainty and, as mentioned earlier, need further documentation and measurement within individual patients and within and across types of strabismus. Both of these observations of sensory behavior can be understood by the sets of macula-periphery, periphery-macula, periphery-periphery, and macula-macula connections the model postulates. It is important to note that normal as well as abnormal connections coexist in these patients which permit the ready (and surprising) adaptations their sensory behaviors present us as clinicians. Without this surfeit of connections, it would be almost impossible for me to conceive of how adaptable, almost plastic, the sensory behavior of the strabismic patient is. It is the very reason why "pinning down" the sensory phenomenology of strabismus has been so frustrating, hence, so little studied.

Localization

Probably no topic has wasted more time and demonstrated more clearly the adage cited at the beginning of this chapter — adaptation to failed comprehension is apathy — than has the subject of correspondence or abnormal correspondence as it is labeled in the strabismus literature. I believe an interesting substudy of the strabismus literature would comprise a simple frequency histogram, by year, of the number of articles since its first description almost a century ago. Still more interesting might be a plot of those articles grouped along a Z axis labeled "theories," for there are many. I do not propose to review them here. That is well done in the cited references. Rather, we turn our attention to the following straightforward predictions derived from the dysconnection theory. First, and most important, the theory predicts that unusual topographic mappings of the central visual field would have to occur as a result of the dysconnections in play under binocular

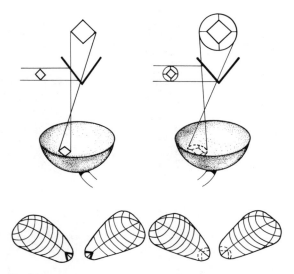

FIGURE 6.10. "Center-surround" effect noted in the behavior of the deviated eye in response to adjustment of the stimulation of the fixing eye. Addition of the circular surround to the stimulus pattern gives rise to suppression of the macula in the deviated eye seen in haploscopic view.

conditions in strabismus (Figure 6.11). If so-called normal correspondence is a by-product of the tight "point-to-point" connections present in the normal visual system, then abnormal correspondence (if you choose to call it that) is a necessary by-product of a set or sets of abnormal connections in the strabismic. It exists in every case of strabismus whether we uncover it or not. It has to. Anatomy gives rise to function as far as this property is concerned. Of what use is it? In my view, none of the reasons advanced make any sense; neither fusion nor avoidance of diplopia, nor adaptation to prevailing conditions, nor provision of a reason for the clinician to perform one of a battery of tests is sufficient reason for anomalous correspondence to exist. The most consistent fact to emerge from any study of the results of sensory testing for abnormal localization is the inconsistency of the test result within and across tests. The most predictable method of altering the behavior of localization is to alter the motor behavior of the strabismic. Inevitably, the localization will change and change in the direction of the change in ocular posture. It may not succeed in adapting completely to that new position but will, with time, move always in that direction. Why does it so behave? First, it is a direct by-product of the anatomy of the system. Second, it provides a topographic map that is absolute for the eyes in an orbital frame of reference, which is the frame of reference necessary to permit the eyes to move freely, accurately, and fully within their respective orbits while freely alternating

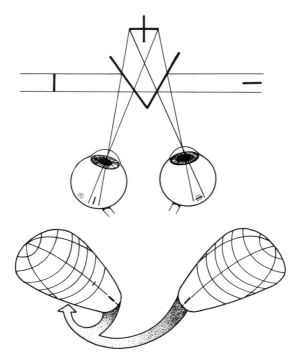

FIGURE 6.11. Connections in the central visual fields of the strabismic give rise to the phenomenology of abnormal localization.

fixation between the eyes in flight. It is this position function in the accurate acquisition of targets moving on the retina that the strabismic does so flawlessly, yet our adult diplopic patient with an acquired deviation of the visual axis and so-called normal correspondence does so poorly and is so distressed by that performance. That is the difference. Strabismics have an extraordinarily accurate map for their saccadic and pursuit systems which makes their function error-free. It is always adapted to where the eyes are, because the location of the eyes is a product of the set of connections in use at the moment. And remember, it is "point-to-field" yet exquisitely accurate at that.

This pattern of localization needs restudy and a fresh look from several points of view. First, we need to look carefully at the areas of the retina in the deviated eye that give responses that are "abnormal" and the areas of the retina that give responses that are "normal" in patients who can be made aware of the phenomenon. Such a mapping is probably the best clinical estimate of the linear extent of the dysconnections existing between the eyes. Second, we need to know what manipulations of motor behavior, other than surgery, will change correspondence. Will manipulation of the accommodative, convergence, optokinetic, and/or vestibular systems change localization behavior? What is the relationship between induced errors of localization (by surgery), so-called paradoxical diplopia, and the postoperative behavior of eye movements? How do these two variables change with respect to each other and over time? How quickly does the new set of dysconnections adapt and stabilize the residual ocular deviation and the localization to permit the strabismic to perform effortlessly as before? These are only a few of the fascinating questions for which the interested clinician will seek meaningful, demystified answers.

If we do as Blake suggests, we might find our view, if not infinite, at least moving in that direction.

7
What Can Studies of Visual Development Tell Us?

As children get older, they get better at things. Whatever it is, girls do it before boys. Everything develops along with everything else.

John McKee's Three Laws of Developmental Psychology

Within my clinical lifetime, an infant science (no pun intended), that of visual development, was conceived, has been born, and is now toddling merrily along. Though its roots go back no longer than my life span in medicine, it has moved out of the descriptive era and begun to develop as a science of measurement and quantification. It incubated as a laboratory science for most of this interval and seemed somewhat remote, addressing questions not terribly important to me, such as binocular acuity development (when I was interested in each eye's vision), thresholds for contrast and color discrimination, and retinal adaptation. If that period was, in retrospect, essential in building an infrastructure of knowledge and training a cadre of investigators who would explore the world outside the laboratory and have the analytical rigor necessary to make quantitative judgments in that world, it was by all means worth it. And as I reflect on this fact, I am aware that I was using the fixation behavior of each eye, granted pitting one against the other was the most crucial part of this experiment, as my *sole* measure of the acuity performance of the infant and preverbal child. In this I was in the company of most of my clinical colleagues. But the world has changed; visual development is now a robust young science, both laboratory and applied. It is no longer tucked away in departments of psychology but is firmly established in the clinic. And quantitative questions such as "Is there one half an octave (20/40 versus 20/60) difference between the acuity of the two eyes with and without this pair of glasses?" are now appropriate. Behind these first-line questions are more sophisticated ones about visual field, stereopsis, and fusion, to which quantitative answers are sought, in my view, and will be found in the next decade or so in the clinic. On another level, still at the stage of laboratory development, are the more elaborate (and costly, though less labor intensive) systems in which the answers to questions of visual performance are teased out by recording brain wave potentials and subjecting the data so obtained to increasingly abstract (and therefore perhaps more susceptible to real error) mathematic analyses, such as Fourier, "fast" Fourier, and extrapolation to zero voltage. These are still firmly laboratory-based devices, requiring as they do the loving care of the Ph.D., and seem several orders of magnitude in complexity and dollars away from our clinical science. Yet one can discern just over the horizon a hybridization of the best of labor-intensive infant "preferential looking" techniques and sophisticated electronic and computer-based recording and analysis of brain potentials that will provide insight into the visual behavior of the neonate, infant, and toddler where we need it most, in the clinic.

Lest my reader feel this chapter too fulsome in its praise of this emerging clinical science, let me hasten to add here a caution: There is, as I see it, a real weakness in the system as it now comes to us. It measures a sensory threshold but it uses a motor behavior to do so. There is a tacit assumption in all of this that if the infant can see it, he or she will look at it. For most purposes this assumption is justified, but I would submit that it is in the clinic where exceptions to this assumption would most likely be encountered, for example, in a complex, multiply handicapped child with delayed maturation of all systems. And it is for these children that valid measures of acuity are most needed.

Where might we begin to use the insights of visual development to help us deepen our understanding of the subject of interest, strabismus. Let us start with the motor behavior of looking at a grating. In line with the logic of the preceding discussion, the motor behavior of the reflex act—that of looking at the grating itself—needs to be explored as scrupulously as the sensory threshold it determines. Although references to "unusual" behaviors on the part of strabismics have been made in passing, no systematic study has attempted to quantitate this behavior. This needs to be described from at least two aspects. The first aspect is the effect of strabismus, if any, on threshold measurements independent of amblyopia and anisometropia. Are strabismic infants any less capable of achieving thresholds considered within the range of normal, even when they are determined to have "normal" vision by clinical testing because they freely alternate? I suspect the answer is yes, or these infants lie at the lower end of the range; this hypothesis is obviously subject to experimental testing. The second aspect is the motor behavior of the strabismic infant looking at the target. What does the saccade to the target look like? Are its parameters (size, acceleration, velocity) normal or within the range of normal? Does the pattern of movement change as the threshold is approached for the strabismic? What does the fixation of the target look like? Obviously the behavior of the normal person in this domain needs to be closely observed as well. I realize that any experimental program in this area necessitates a shift in emphasis in the world of infant testing from strictly threshold measurements to an enlarged arena in which thresholds are viewed not only as levels of resolution attained but as the manner in which those levels were attained as well. Threshold determinations are then seen as complex sensorimotor acts that are in themselves a manifestation of the development of the central nervous system. What is the motor strategy adopted by the "normal" eye(s) of the normal infant as opposed to the "normal" eye(s) of the strabismic infant? To me, the science is now mature enough and the threshold measure secure enough that such second-order questions can and should be raised not only for their own intrinsic value but also to keep this science growing in a clinically biased direction.

Also requiring further evaluation are the fascinating reports of Aslin, Archer, and their colleagues on the results of infant testing for stereopsis employing a modification of the random dot–OKN (optokinetic nystagmus) stripe paradigm. They reported no evidence of preoperative responses suggesting stereopsis in a group of congenital esotropic patients; immediately after surgery, presumably when the visual axes were aligned, stereo behavior began to emerge that was subsequently lost within a matter of weeks, presumably when the visual axes redeviated. The conventional explanation of the phenomenon would invoke passive loss of the stereo function as a result of misalignment of the visual axes. I would suggest another interpretation of the phenomenon—active competition between several neuronal networks all competing for dominance of the motor output apparatus after a surgical alignment procedure. No one alignment position (network) clearly carries the highest "information" during this period as far as the visual brain is concerned. Any or all therapeutic interventions during this phase of plasticity designed to support the network we identify as "normal" may, in fact, be decisive.

A rerun of this experimental paradigm as a "thought experiment" might proceed as follows: Immediately after surgery, stereo thresholds are attainable and the infants' eyes appear aligned within the limits imposed by the inherent "noise" in measurements of this type. Thresholds are recorded more than once a day up to the infant's tolerance by employing videographics, cartoons, colors, and movements to sustain interest, as a therapeutic as well as a diagnostic measure. Day 2 and 3 stereo thresholds begin to fall without obvious deviation of the visual axes. A potential explanation is that a "coarser"-grained network is being employed on a trial-and-error provisional basis by the central nervous system. Intervention here might call for spectacles to correct any refractive error (postoperative astigmatism?); prisms, if any shift in ocular posture is noted; or patches, if suspending binocular vision seems the only intervention possible. Diagnosis and therapy are resumed on a daily basis until the stereo thresholds are reestablished and stabilized. Oculinum therapy might be employed to correct any small misalignments if they are thought to be beyond the reach of prisms. The point here is to manipulate the visual environment in such a way as to support bimacular stimulation until stabilization. End of thought experiment.

What is envisioned here is a cooperative undertaking by the clinical and developmental scientist that is part experiment, part therapy (goal-directed activity). Obviously, one of the outcomes could be failure, but we already know that as a possible outcome. Archer et al. reported 100% loss of the stereo behavior and recurrence of abnormal ocular posture in their infants. I suggest that with a different conceptualization of the underlying central nervous system mechanism, there emerge a rather different meaning and a strategy for dealing with this rather well-known postoperative motor behavior. We simply do not know if stereo behavior might be present in many or all of those children, yet the theory predicts that it should be. It is not my purpose to delve into or develop therapeutic measures to be tested. Rather, my purpose is to point out an area worthy of scientific study to bring together the visual scientist and a clinician in the arena of strabismus and strabismus behaviors both pre- and postoperatively.

Yet a third area suggests itself as an agenda item for visual development, the prodromal behavior of the strabismic. What developmental clues might make us suspect that a neonate, infant, or toddler is likely to develop strabismus? Obviously, observation of such behavior patterns, if present, would be of immense importance to possible prevention, early diagnosis, and/or therapy, none of which is of direct concern to us here. Let us instead turn our attention to how we might identify a population and begin searching for such behaviors. The most logical place/time to start would be birth and the most logical population to start with would be an "enriched" sample: our own strabismic patient population. For purposes of such study, every pregnancy that occurs within a family with one or more strabismic members would be considered an "at risk" pregnancy. Pregnancy history should be carefully scrutinized and any deviation from the norm recorded, with its significance to be judged later. The object of our interest though is the newborn and her or his earliest developing visuomotor behavior patterns. Scanning eye movements, eye contact, fixation, REM sleep, and changes in alignment over time are a few of these patterns. Acuity, monocularly and binocularly, and the motor behaviors manifested by the infant, particularly those at or around threshold, would seem to be prime subjects of study. Abnormal persistence of immature oculomotor behavior patterns such as flutter, dysmetria, and other identified patterns should be sought for as well. Care should be taken in the interpretation of all of the perinatal data to include suitable weighting and adjustment according to difficulty and complications of labor and delivery and the type and quantity of anesthesia and narcotic agent(s) employed.

Moving forward in time, the first well-baby exam (6 weeks) might also serve as a survey of visual functions and behaviors. Even if strabismus does not develop in a particular infant in a family, valuable normative data will begin to accumulate within these pedigrees that can, in turn, serve as the standard against which abnormal behaviors can be measured. Why am I emphasizing the data-gathering expedition, which is obviously labor and time intensive? Because, very simply, I do not believe that strabismus arises "ex machina"; rather I believe it arises in the context of a vast developmental program which, unfolding before the eye of the critical observer, fits together as pieces of a puzzle with what comes before and what follows after. Stressing the system with threshold measurements seems, to me, to be the most direct means of finding its abnormalities, if any. There may exist other, more subtle strategies by which these behavior patterns could be observed. Using an enriched sample, that is, newborns of strabismic families, as the initial subjects recommends itself to me because of the high likelihood of finding defects, if any are to be found. There is also the intriguing possibility of recognizing in the offspring of these families *para*strabismic sensory and motor behaviors, which, though they do not result in the frank clinical syndrome, nevertheless cannot be classified as normal. Tracking such behaviors over time in this group might help explain such later-life problems as clumsiness, poor hand and eye coordination, reading and learning difficulties, and visual perception problems. Though I do not set forth these speculations as a formal testable hypothesis here, observations of early visuomotor behavior, particularly abnormalities, may prove helpful in conceptualizing the mechanisms by which later maladaptive behaviors manifest, when the child begins to play ball, write, and read.

As I look forward I see, perhaps in the next decade, the development of a robust science based on cooperation between visual and clinical specialists who expend their effort on a subject of profound interest to both—the strabismic infant as an experiment of nature, of great magnitude and sophistication—to penetrate beneath the surface phenomena and understand, at the deepest level possible, the developing nervous system involved.

8
How Can Visual Psychophysics Help Us?

It is function that breathes life into anatomy and perception that vivifies sensory electro-physiology.

W.A.H. Rushton

There is perhaps no field in the human biosciences that approaches as closely the physical sciences, in terms of rigor of hypothesis testing and exactitude of measurement, as does visual psychophysics. This has been its tradition since its birth in the last century with Purkinje, Weber, Helmholtz, Hering, and Sherrington. If for no other reason than their rigor and discipline, it is essential that visual psychophysicists become deeply involved in the noninvasive study of the clinical phenomenology of strabismus. Thus far, the number of psychophysicists involved has been small but their contributions have been of major importance. It is not my purpose to review these here in detail. Suffice it to say that reading their work has convinced me of the need to engage them more fully in our clinical problem, strabismus.

In this chapter, I present several questions. Though I do not know them, the answers to these questions have important bearing on our knowledge of the three central phenomena of strabismus: inhibition of information in the central visual field of the deviated eye, anomalous localization in this field, and a defect in ocular posture. As I made clear earlier, I believe all three are simply different manifestations of the same basic defect—the dysconnection state of the visual nervous system. If this is so, certain effects should be observed under static and dynamic conditions in the strabismic that are not observed in the normal person.

My first question concerns visual "space" as mapped in the central visual field of the fixing eye. Because of the process of alternation between the eyes, I believe the dysconnections are always reciprocal and that information flows in both directions at all times (Figure 8.1). Traffic flowing from the deviated eye to the fixing eye is easily handled by inhibition mechanisms in this eye so that it never reaches conscious awareness. Yet it represents information that might produce a distortion in the spatial map of the central visual field of the fixing eye in some very specific ways; for example, it might result in the surface of an object in space

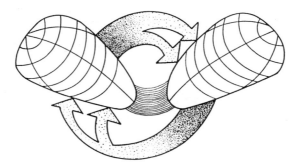

FIGURE 8.1. The reciprocal nature of the dysconnections between the macula of the fixing eye and the periphery of the deviated eye.

being perceived as smaller than it should be because of a "field-point" effect (Figure 8.2). The key here is to realize that the surface "raster" in the nervous system by which real objects in space are visualized is a composite of the rasters of the two eyes, in the case of strabismus, a fine macular raster for the fixing eye and a coarser peripheral raster for the deviated eye. Both, however, together provide a subjective metric for the visual surface. Obviously, the other eye could not be used as a control because the defect would be replicated in this eye as well. It seems that normal observers with similar refractive errors and normal fusion, stereopsis, and oculomotor behavior would be necessary for testing. Though the effect may be slight, it should be there if it is sought. It is important also in choosing a strabismic subject to be sure that alternation is free and acuity and refractive error are equal. The alternation does not have to be 50/50 but should not require a cover test to produce it. I realize that in proposing this test, I am implying that the "packing density" of visual connections somehow plays a role in our spatial metric. I believe it does. I do not believe that the test array should be a ruler or a metric scale because the ruler itself may be distorted in its horizontal (and perhaps vertical) dimensions. Rather, the test stimulus array must be something more subtle and elegant, perhaps some comparison of like surfaces for equality of area. In any case, I leave that question to the psychophysicists; clearly they are the masters of this domain.

My next question concerns the properties of the central visual field of the deviated eye. One cannot help but wonder at the ease with which, someplace in the visual system, the bulk of the information in the central visual field of the deviated eye is edited and how very precisely so. Literally in the blink of an eye, or even without that blink, the fixation will change between eyes and the formerly deviated eye will assume fixation. Its central visual field, dominated by the macula, will see normally and not a trace of suppression of information will remain. Or does it? As the reader knows, I have once again relied on dysconnections to serve as an explanation for this switching behavior. But what is the

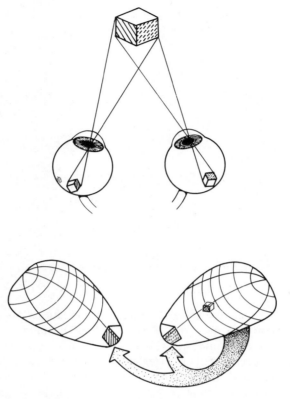

FIGURE 8.2. The abnormal spatial perception that might be observed in strabismus because of the very different "spatial raster" employed by the strabismic in binocular vision.

mechanism by which inhibition works? Two alternatives come to mind. The first is an inhibitory mechanism by which the threshold in the deviated eye is elevated so that for all ordinary photopic and scotopic luminances, all visual objects in this central visual field are below threshold. According to the second or "noise" hypothesis, the information flowing from the macula of the fixing eye is such a dense and noisy signal to the central visual field of the deviated eye that all "real" signals are drowned by it (Figure 8.3). As a clinician, I am inclined toward the latter because of a common clinical observation: When I dim the illumination to the central visual fields of both eyes, simplify the signal to a single light point, and, for instance, introduce a slight difference in stimulus quality — a light red filter before the fixing eye — I can almost always elicit diplopia in the alternating strabismic. In my simple understanding of the matter, I have, by manipulating the variables in the central visual field of the fixing eye, made this signal less "noisy" and therefore permitted the signal in the central visual field of the deviated eye

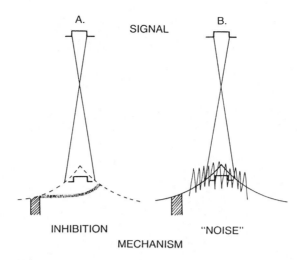

FIGURE 8.3. Inhibition versus the "noise" hypothesis resulting in a blanking of visual objects in the central visual field of the deviated eye in strabismics.

to emerge. I realize that this may not be a valid interpretation of the phenomenon from the standpoint of the psychophysicist. It is therefore all the more important that by designing and executing a critical experimental test or tests, we should be able to decide between these alternatives. Why is it so important? Because it goes to the very nature of the defect in strabismus, which is, as I conceive it, an over-abundance of innervation rather than a lack of innervation or an "inhibition" causing a loss of information.

The third question concerns another property of the scotoma in the central visual field of the strabismic subject, its "behavior at the boundary." My concept of the scotoma in strabismus is that it is governed very much by a sort of Heisenberg's uncertainty principle—the scotoma appears to us, the observers, to be very much influenced by how we observe it. It changes as we change the conditions under which we test for it. Obviously if we search for it under monocular conditions, it appears to be gone without a trace. And that is an important clue to its behavior. If, now, we present a single point of light as a fixation target for the fixing eye and search for the scotoma in the central visual field of the deviated eye separated haploscopically from its fellow, the scotoma will appear small and central, if we see it at all in this eye. If we employ targets with increased dimensions, contours, and contrasts in the central visual field of the fixing eye, the scotoma plotted in the central visual field of the deviated eye will expand. What variables control this expansion? Are they spatial? Are they contour or luminance driven? Are there other variables (Figure 8.4)? In effect, this calls for measuring the extent and nature of a process in the deviated eye by changing the signal in both eyes until one of two endpoints is reached: diplopia or a shift in fixation. Obviously, the targets for the two eyes would have to be different enough that we could

A. LUMINANCE   B. CONTOUR

C. SPATIAL

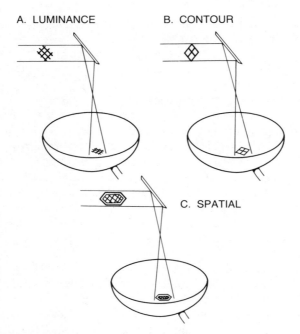

FIGURE 8.4. Changes in stimulus luminance, contour, or size resulting in expansion of the area of suppression in the central visual field of the deviated eye.

be sure the target for the deviated eye was, in fact, invisible to this eye until it reached some sort of threshold. A second requirement of such an experiment would be careful monitoring of both eyes for movement. The reason for this is that part of the strategy adapted by the dysconnection state is to employ small eye movements to maintain the visual world stable.

A second important variable that might be measured by this sort of experimental paradigm involves a question that has bedeviled clinical measurements in strabismus—the question of "central" and "peripheral." In clinical lexicon, "central" refers loosely to macula ("fovea to fovea" being a special case), about 5° of the central visual field centered on the fovea of the deviated eye. "Peripheral" refers to areas beyond that. Thus, clinicians speak of "cures," for example, after alignment of the visual axes within 5° of one another at a given testing distance. Within that range "central fusion" (not fovea-to-fovea fusion) may occur; beyond that range one can only hope for "peripheral fusion" to occur. Is there any basis for this parcellation of the central visual field? If there is, then presumably it should be possible to map behavior at its boundary and some change of state should occur from one to another. Further, it might be predicted that within the central or macular region, motor behavior might be insensitive to stimulus change, whereas, in the peripheral zone, motor behavior might begin to develop, signaling an attempt to adapt the ocular posture to incoming sensory information either to inhibit this target signal in the deviated eye, to shift fixation, or to make a dysjugate movement to align target contours. In any case, the results of such experiments performed under careful sensory and motor control would shed a good deal of light on the nature and behavior of inhibition in the central visual field of the deviated eye under static conditions.

The next questions relate to "visuomotor behavior under dynamic conditions." The eyes are, after all, our most mobile sense organ and, in fact, are built to avoid static conditions. They are practically never still, always seeking to renew the visual scene and fill it with new and interesting objects. Turning to our strabismic model, it seems reasonable to ask three questions related to localization. First, how does our strabismic steer the eyes in a very special set of circumstances, when shifting fixation from one to the other eye? Having observed many strabismic children performing this task effortlessly and some fewer adults performing this test with considerable difficulty, I can testify that there is a difference. I do not believe it resides in simply the presence of diplopia in the adults and its absence in the children.

This first experiment, really a series of experiments, would be designed to test the type of localization the strabismic employs when performing saccadic and pursuit eye movements. The dysconnection theory predicts that because of the nature of these connections, abnormalities of localization, although present in the strictest sense, are perfectly adapted to the deviation of the visual axes. In fact, they are in register and exist to provide that adaptation to the deviation. "Normal correspondence" is defined operationally in the normal subject by a set of "normal anatomical connections." In the case of strabismus, "normal correspondence" is maintained by a set of connections between anatomically disparate yet connected points in the binocular visual field. The theory postulates that because of these connections, normal relationships are maintained within subjective visual space. If this is true, the central visual field of the deviated eye maintains a perfectly congruent map of spatial values aligned with those of the fixing eye but transposed to the peripheral visual field of the deviated eye. And it is this congruent coordinate system that is responsible for the flawless shift of fixation between the two. The experimental paradigm employed to test this hypothesis would be very much like that employed by Robinson in investigating the dynamics of the saccadic system and is as follows: With both eyes performing programmed pursuit or saccadic eye movements led by the fixing eye, a target to be fixed is delivered off axis to the deviated eye, subthreshold and haploscopically. The strabismic subject is instructed to fix this new target whenever its presence is signaled, by an auditory clue perhaps. The theory predicts that the subject would make an errorless shift in fixation to the stationary (saccadic mode) or moving (pursuit mode) but consciously unseen target. If the correspondence is "normal" in the strict definition, the subject would make an error equal to the size of the angle of the deviation between the visual axes. If the correspondence is abnormal but not adapted to the deviation between the two visual axes, the subject would make an error less than the first error but not zero. If the correspondence is normal in the sense of fully adapted to a "normal-by-virtue-of-connections" state, the error would be zero. The behavior discussed here is the very flexible, yet fully in register, state in which these dysconnections place the central visual field of the strabismic eye. It is, in fact, behavior that in some senses mimics the utrocular behavior of the reptilian and amphibian visual systems so beautifully described by Walls. These systems are totally decussated yet coordinated.

The next experimental paradigm is similar to the preceding one, but measures the effects on the localization behavior of the deviated eye of influencing the accommodative system by means of minus and plus lenses and of influencing the vestibular system by means of Bárány chair rotation—two very different manipulations of the sensorimotor system. Once again, the theory predicts that the dysconnection would be robust and would maintain perfect topographic alignment in spite of the manipulations, as demonstrated by the error-free shift in fixation to a subthreshold target presented haploscopically in the deviated eye.

The final experiments are designed to test another prediction that has up to now been implicit, but unstated: normal and abnormal connections coexist in the dysconnection state. The experimental paradigm is similar to that employed previously but the signal is delivered, once again by means of haploscopic device, subthreshold at the moving macula of the deviated eye. The prediction would be an error-free shift to take up fixation. The key to understanding this apparent paradox is to conceptualize correspondence as a very plastic phenomenon that depends for its existence and metric on the connections stimulated and in play at any given moment.

In summary then, in this chapter we have examined a number of experiments that call for the rigor and discipline so typical of this learned profession of psychophysics, yet turned now to a clinical problem that is in essence of surpassing interest: How does the visual system process information along the domain of space and time and motion? The system presented for study is, in many respects, quite close to the normal but, in other respects, quite different. That is the essence of the challenge.

Horace Barlow, in another context, quoted an otherwise unnamed "eminent neurophysiologist" to the effect that "while neurophysiology is exciting, it is likely to be wrong while psychophysics, though dull, is likely to be right." I hope that pyschophysicists will invest their considerable talents and insights in one of nature's most fascinating experiments, strabismus.

9
How Can Studies of Overall Development Help Us?

Passing hence from infancy, I came to boyhood, or rather it came to me, displacing infancy. Nor did that depart—(for whither went it?) and yet it is no more.

St. Augustine

The milieu in which I see strabismus occurring is critical not only for the development of the visual system but also for the global development of the fetus and neonate as well. My goal in this chapter is to enlarge the circle of phenomenology we must carefully examine if we are to place strabismus in its true perspective. It is not a thing apart. It happens in time and to a developing human being. A before and an after and, if I am not mistaken, a "something else" accompany it. I come to this conclusion on at least two grounds. The first is a consideration of the central hypothesis, which postulates a specific time, site, and mechanism by which an insult is delivered to the developing visual system. Synaptogenesis in its decrescendo (dying back) phase is implicated. But synaptogenesis, as has been pointed out, is a systemwide process occurring in all cortical areas on almost the same schedule. Though not intuitively obvious, this simultaneity (of synaptogenesis) does make sense from the standpoint of having much of the central nervous system circuitry and all primary areas of sensory and motor processing ready as early as possible before, during, or slightly after birth. What this means is that we should then look at the other special senses, at the somasthetic and motor behavior and, yes, even early cognition and learning, for evidence of a unique clinical entity, "global synaptic plethora," that might result in the production or survival of primitive motor and sensory behavior patterns long after they should normally disappear. Or, on the other hand, more advanced and integrated motor, sensory, or even cognitive behaviors might be delayed in appearance as a result of this dysmorphology of synapses. Although strabismus is the central phenomenon we observe as a result of this process, the very nature of the defect in the process—the failure of synapses to die back—would predict patterns of observable abnormal behavior outside the visual system. A second consideration leads in the same direction. Strabismus is found as a part of almost every type of developmental condition, be it the result of trauma, inflammation, or genetic or metabolic insult; if a neurodevelopmental insult occurs beyond the stage that gives rise to major organ malformations but still early enough, strabismus is its inevitable companion. A caution here: I do not seek, in any of these entities, "a cause" or "the cause" of strabismus. We have carefully avoided any linkage between well-defined dysmorphology syndromes, whatever their basis (genetic, epigenetic, or a combination), and our model of strabismus. Far too many cases of strabismus, sui generis, occur without any obvious stigma of those syndromes to implicate them as a causal mechanism. Rather, I see strabismus as almost an aftereffect of a far more fundamental and devastating change that gives rise to the dysmorphic syndrome itself. The point is not a trivial one. We are searching for small-scale, subtle clues in an overall central nervous system development plan that will accompany our prototypical strabismus model, not gross, obvious clues that clamor for our attention. Our efforts then are those of the detective, not the cop on the beat.

In Utero

Let us briefly review what is known about the period of development that concerns us and cast our questions in the light of this knowledge. Ultrasound has given us an entirely new concept of what the fetus is capable of at different stages of development and it is here that we should start our search.

Seventh-month: Most reflex response patterns are established. Crying, breathing, swallowing, and sucking are apparent in the child's in utero behavior.

Eighth-month: The fetus weighs between 5 and 7 pounds and, because of cramped living conditions, its movements are reduced.

Ninth-month: The fetus approaches term after having been in the womb 260 to 270 days. Heart rate speeds up.

In utero, signs of other systems' involvement might take the form of delayed development of the postural, sucking, crying, or breathing reflexes which, although they do not begin in this era, nevertheless reach their peak of intrauterine development here. We might hypothesize that just as strabismus represents an atavistic preservation of connections impeding full development of binocular vision, so a persistence of connections might well hinder or slow development of reflex behavior patterns in other sensory, motor, and associative areas. The design of an experiment to test this hypothesis in utero is not at once obvious; however, preliminary studies may be made of pregnant women with family histories positive for strabismus. In utero milestones of development, including the onset and development of eye movements, might be delayed. Care would have to be taken to exclude other sources of central nervous system pathology and to follow the offspring studied intensively in utero, both at birth and during infancy, for evidence of the development of strabismus along with other abnormal sensory and motor reflex patterns.

TABLE 9.1. Major neonatal reflexes.

Reflex	Formulation of stimulation	Response	Developmental course	Significance
Optical or acoustic reflex	Shine bright light suddenly at infant's eyes, or clap hands 30 cm from infant's head	Quick closure of eyelids	Permanent	Protection from strong stimulation; absent in some infants with impaired visual or auditory systems
Tonic neck reflex	Turn head to one side while infant lies awake on back	Infant assumes a "fencing posture"; arm is extended on side toward which head is turned; opposite arm is flexed with the hand resting near or in the head-chest region	Characteristic of the first 12 weeks, but is not consistently present; fades by the 16th week	If constantly present, may indicate neurological dysfunction
Biceps reflex	Tap on tendon of biceps muscle in elbow area	Short contraction of biceps muscle	Brisker in the first 2 days of life than later	Absent in depressed infants or in cases of congenital muscular disease
Knee jerk	Tap on tendon just below the knee	Quick extension of the knee	More pronounced during first 2 days of life than later	Absent or difficult to obtain in depressed infants or in cases of congenital muscular disease
Palmar grasp reflex	Place finger into infant's hand and press against palmar surface	Spontaneous grasp of examiner's finger	Less intense during first 2 days of life than later; disappears at 3 to 4 months of age	Absent or difficult to obtain in depressed infants; facilitated by sucking movements
Babinski reflex	Stroke sole of infant's foot from toes toward heel	Extension of big toe and spreading of smaller toes	Disappears between 8 months and 1 year	Absent in infants with defects of the lower spinal cord
Withdrawal reflex	Prick soles of foot with a pin	Withdrawal, with flexion of foot, knee, and hip	Constantly present during first 10 days; weaker thereafter	Protection from unpleasant tactile stimulation; absent in infants with defects of the lower spinal cord; weakened by breech birth and sciatic nerve damage

Reflex	Stimulation	Response		
Rooting reflex	Tickle skin at one corner of mouth	Head turns toward source of stimulation; infant tries to suck the stimulating finger	Less vigorous during the first 2 days; most readily elicited in infants 1 to 2 weeks old; disappears by 3 weeks as it becomes a voluntary head-turning response	Assists baby in finding nipple; absent in depressed infants
Sucking reflex	Place index finger 3 to 4 cm into mouth	Head turns toward source of stimulation; infant tries to suck the stimulating finger	Less intense and regular during the first 3 to 4 days	Permits feeding; weak or absent in depressed infants
Moro reflex	Support body horizontally and allow the head to drop a few centimeters, or make a sudden loud sound or bang on the surface supporting the infant	Back arches, baby extends legs and throws arms outward and then in toward the midline of the body, as if to grab on for support	Disappears by the middle of the first year	Absent or weak Moro indicates serious disturbances of the central nervous system
Walking reflex	Hold infant under arms and permit bare feet to touch a flat surface	Infant lifts one foot after another in walking response	Generally disappears by 8 weeks; retained longer in babies who are lighter in weight and if the reflex is exercised	May be absent in infants born by breech presentation and in depressed infants

Adapted from Laura E. Berk, *Child Development*. Copyright © 1989 by Allyn and Bacon. After Prechtl and Beintema (1965); Knobloch and Pasamanick (1974). Used with permission.

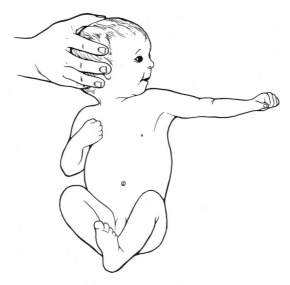

FIGURE 9.1. Fencing or tonic neck position reflex.

Birth and the Puerperium

It is unlikely that clues to the development of other central nervous system abnormalities will be found in the newborn's Apgar score or gross neurological evaluation. Had the developmental abnormality been so gross as to produce defects at this level, it would have long since been obvious to all. Nor is it likely that conditions such as respiratory distress syndrome and intraventricular hemorrhage, conditions that affect primarily the premature neonate, are likely to provide clues. Although the incidence of strabismus is higher in premature neonates, I believe that its basis is other than what we seek.

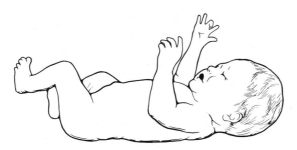

FIGURE 9.2. Moro reflex.

FIGURE 9.3. Plantar grasp reflex.

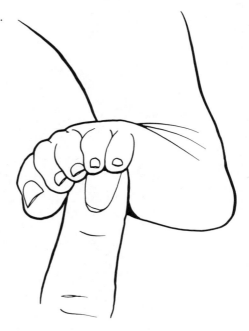

Reflexes of the Newborn

See Table 9.1.

We now turn our attention to such examples of reflex behavior as the asymmetric tonic neck reflex or fencing position reflex (appearance: 24 to 28 weeks of gestation; disappearance: 12 to 18 weeks after birth) (Figure 9.1). The Moro reflex (28 weeks of gestation 4 to 6 weeks after birth) is another potential marker (Figure 9.2), not with respect to its appearance but for its *disappearance*, which is obviously a part of programmed motor development. Disappearance of the neck righting reflex (34 to 36 weeks of gestation to 12 weeks after birth), the traction reflex (32 to 36 weeks of gestation to 4 to 6 months after birth when control of the neck becomes volitional) and the tonic labyrinthine reflex, which also disappears by 4 to 6 months of age, is of interest to us. The positive supporting reflex, the stepping reaction, the placing reflex, the plantar grasp reflex (Figure 9.3), and the Babinsky reflex (Figure 9.4) span the period of interest to us. The theory would predict that some or all of these reflex behaviors, which are a normal part of the infant's developmental repertoire, would persist beyond the time they should disappear. The pattern of persistence may, in fact, be an important clue as to when the insult occurred.

Behavioral States

Sleep, drowsiness, alertness, and crying are four other areas to which our inquiry should extend. Seven categories of the newborn's behavior have been described

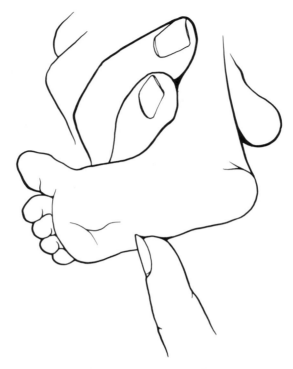

FIGURE 9.4. Babinsky reflex.

(Table 9.2). These need to be systemically studied for evidence of abnormal parcellation of the neonate's time. A group that might best be studied first is infants with early-onset strabismus (first 2 to 6 months of life) versus normal controls.

Other Senses

Touch is present at birth. There is a specific patterned motor response to both touch and pain. The latter is a withdrawal response.

Hearing constitutes an interesting test of our hypothesis. Once amniotic fluid is drained from the ears at birth, the neonate probably has the auditory acuity of adults. Low-frequency sounds, whispers, lullabies, metronomes, and heartbeat all calm the neonate. High-frequency sounds arouse the neonate. The auditory evoked potential at birth should be normal and should provide some clue as to what extent the auditory system participates, if it does, in this abnormal process. It is so close to vision as a special sense, yet because the in utero environment transmits both sounds and gravitational stimuli, it develops so much earlier than does vision, that one would suspect that it might be spared.

TABLE 9.2. Newborn states.

Regular sleep	The infant is at full rest and shows little or no diffuse motor activity. The eyelids are closed, no spontaneous eye movements occur, and the facial muscles are in repose. The rate and depth of respiration are even and regular.
Periodic sleep	This state is intermediate between regular and irregular sleep. The infant shows slightly more motor activity than in regular sleep. Respiratory movements are periodic; bursts of rapid, shallow breathing alternate with bursts of deep, slow respiration.
Irregular sleep	Motor activity is greater than in periodic sleep and varies from gentle limb movements to occasional stirring. Facial grimaces and mouthing occur, and occasional rapid eye movements can be observed through the eyelids. The rate and depth of respiration are irregular, and breathing occurs at a generally faster pace than it does in regular sleep.
Drowsiness	In this state, the infant is either falling asleep or waking up. The baby is less active than in periodic or irregular sleep, but more active than in regular sleep. Eyes open and close intermittently. When open, they have a glazed appearance and are poorly focused. When the infant is waking up, spurts of gross motor activity tend to occur. Respiration is usually even but somewhat quicker than during regular sleep.
Alert inactivity	The infant is relatively inactive, with eyes open, attentive, and focused. Respiration is constant in frequency and depth.
Waking activity	The infant shows frequent bursts of diffuse motor activity of the limbs, trunk, and head. The face may be relaxed, or tense and wrinkled as if the infant is about to cry, and respiration is very irregular.
Crying	Crying is accompanied by diffuse, vigorous motor activity.

Reproduced, with permission, from Wolff PH. *The Causes, Controls and Organization of Behavior in the Neonate.* New York: International Universities Press; 1966. (Psychological Issues, Vol. 5, No. 1, Monograph 17.)

Smell allows the neonate to discriminate between mother's breast milk and other breast milk. A withdrawal response to ammonia and vinegar is also part of the neonate's repertoire.

Withdrawal from sour-tasting stimuli and puckering in response to sweet-tasting stimuli are typical of the neonate's motor response.

Infancy

The final period of concern to us is infancy. This period extends from 28 days to 1 year of age.

Motor Development

In this period, motor development is quite striking and probably parallels the development of the nervous system. This state of physical maturation is often called *readiness*. The developmental program enables the infant to hold the head up, to crawl, to walk, and finally, to run. It involves maturation of head control,

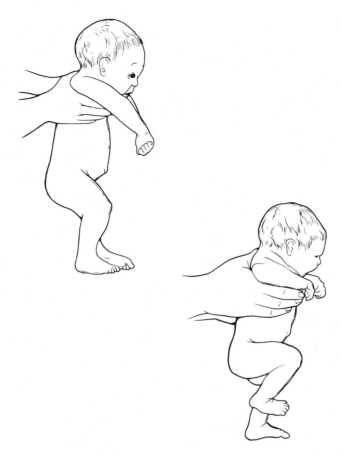

FIGURE 9.5. Sequence of motor development that results in walking by 15 months of age.

posture, sitting, kneeling, crawling, and standing. Walking is generally achieved by 15 months of age and there is a definite sequence to the process (Figure 9.5).

Directed Reach and Grasping

During infancy, children learn to reach toward objects and pick them up. This, too, involves the infants' learning a sequence of movements. The young infant begins by moving the arms in the direction of the object of interest without grasping it. The infant visually monitors the task. Grasping that occurs in the first 2 to 3 months of life is primarily reflexive, but the voluntary grasping that begins at 3 months is prehensile and progresses until the infant uses the entire hand to

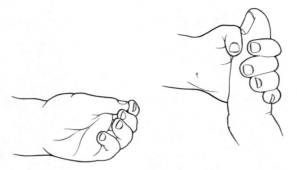

FIGURE 9.6. Pincer grasp.

grasp the object (5 to 7 months). The infant then progresses to a palmar grasp at 9 to 10 months of age and a thumb and forefinger (pincer) grasp at 9 to 15 months (Figure 9.6). Letting go is an equally complex task and it begins at about 7 months of age. The efficient use of two hands begins at 5 to 7 months. By 8 to 10 months the infant can perform independent activity with two hands, for example, supporting body weight with one hand while reaching for objects with the other. Hand preference, however, is not apparent usually until 8 to 9 months of age.

Perception

In the area of perception, most of the science has been concentrated on vision but certain other areas are also important. Early work suggested that at 2 months, infants prefer to look at a "real face" over a "scrambled face" (Figure 9.7). (I believe this capacity is present much earlier.) Other work seems to indicate that at 1 to 2 months of age, infants can scan the outer edges of a face, but at about 5 to 7 weeks, infants begin to make eye contact and thereafter spend more time looking at eyes than faces.

Hearing

As noted earlier, infants are born with the ability to discriminate high- and low-frequency sounds, to adapt to sounds and filter them out, and to attempt to locate sound sources. Infants not only hear well and attend the sounds of a human voice, but also synchronize their body movements to patterns of adult speech. This synchronization is called "language dance." Between 3 and 6 months of age infants can imitate a variety of low- and high-pitched sounds and, by 4 months, can discriminate their parents' voices and distinguish these voices from those of strangers.

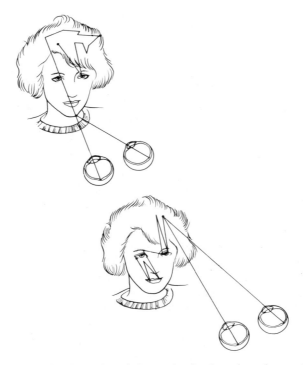

FIGURE 9.7. Visual search an infant makes in observing a human face.

Other Senses

Touch is probably the best developed sense. This is probably why wrapping a neonate or an infant in a blanket and holding him or her have a calming effect. By 1 year of age infants can recognize objects by feel and distinguish common objects by touch in the dark.

Infant Routines

The neonate sleeps 17 to 20 hours per day. By 1 year, infants have slept more than half their extrauterine life. Newborns spend more than 50% of their time in rapid eye movement (REM) sleep, whereas adults spend less than 25% of their time in REM sleep. It is hypothesized that REM sleep may, in fact, be an aid to central nervous system development, and as the infant becomes more alert and aware of environmental stimuli, the need for REM sleep diminishes.

Table 9.3 summarizes the milestones for normal sensorimotor development.

TABLE 9.3. Milestones in sensorimotor development.

Age	Sensorimotor achievements	Vocalization and language
3 months	Grasps objects, smiles spontaneously, holds head steady when sitting, lifts up head when on stomach, follows object readily with eyes	Squeals, coos especially in response to social interaction, laughs
4½ months	Reaches awkwardly for some objects that he sees, frequently looks at hands, readily brings objects in hand to mouth, holds head steady in most positions, sits with props, bears some weight on legs	Seems to search with eyes for speaker, mixes some consonants in with cooing sounds, begins babbling
6 months	Usually reaches for near objects that she sees and looks at objects that she grasps, sits without support leaning forward on hands, bears weight on legs but must be balanced by adult, brings feet to mouth when lying on back	Babbles simple sounds like "mamama" and "bababa," turns to voice, laughs easily
9 months	Grasps small objects with thumb and fingertips, shows first preference for one hand (usually the right), sits upright with good control, stands holding on, crawls, often imitates	Commonly repeats sounds in babbling, produces some intonation patterns of parents' language, imitates some sounds, understands "no"
1 year	Neatly grasps small objects, stands alone, walks with one hand held by adult, seats self on floor, mouths objects much less, drinks from cup but messily, often imitates simple behaviors, cooperates in dressing	Produces a few words such as "mama" and "dada," understands a few simple words and commands, produces sentence-like intonation patterns called expressive jargon
1½ years	Puts cubes in bucket, dumps contents from bottle, walks alone and falls only rarely, uses spoon with little spilling, undresses self, scribbles spontaneously	Produces between 5 and 50 single words, produces complex intonation patterns, understands many words and simple sentences
2 years	Turns single pages in a book, builds tower of blocks, shifts easily between sitting and standing, runs, throws and kicks ball, washes hands, puts on clothing	Produces more than 50 words, produces a few short "sentences," understands much in concrete situations, shows much interest in language and communication

Reproduced, with permission, from Fischer KW, Lazerson A. *Human Development: From Conception Through Adolescence.* New York: WH Freeman; 1984. After Frankenburg and Dodds, 1967; Ilg, Ames, and Baker, 1981; Knoblock and Pasamanick, 1974; Lenneberg, 1967; Ramsay, 1984

Summary

The task before us is in one sense simple and in another complex. We must first identify a cohort or population of infants at risk and study them prospectively to determine at what age they achieve the milestones of (other) sensory, motor, and cognitive development and integration. Gross or marked changes in these other areas would not be expected. In fact, the changes would probably be subtle and reflected in comments made by parents and/or grandparents: "he was always a clumsy (or hyper) baby"; "she was a slow developer"; "he didn't seem as interested as my other baby in his environment." The visual system though occupies the center stage in the developmental drama during this period and defects there are the ones resulting in strabismus, whereas defects in other sensory, motor, and integrative systems that mature later (after the effect of the insult has dissipated?) are likely to be less affected and the evidence for them more difficult to discern. Nevertheless, development is a wondrous symphony and all of its movements must be heard. By putting strabismus right in the center of this developmental context, we begin to learn, I believe, more about it and the overall process of development as well. This is the path to the answer to the question posed at the beginning of the chapter.

10
What Can the Imaging Technology of the Central Nervous System Tell Us?

And other spirits there are standing apart
Upon the forehead of the age to come;
These will give the world another heart
And other pulses. Hear ye not the hum?
Of mighty workings in the human mart?
Listen awhile ye nations, and be dumb.

John Keats

Goethe, the great poet and natural scientist, raised a fundamental objection to the way that science was done in his time: "The isolation of phenomenon and processes from their natural environment to permit their analysis and understanding, does violence to the object studied and changes its real nature." His objection remains as valid today as when he made it. Yet science has not paused to answer it. It was and is the only path visible to us. Yet if one views developments in the field of imaging of the central nervous system and its activity in the broadest sense, we are coming closer and closer to the ideal of the poet—that of studying natural phenomena in their natural habitat. In our case, the object of interest is the human nervous system and its development. The techniques we speak of in this chapter are images of one type or another of the form and function of that nervous system.

Under "images," as used in this chapter, I group recording of the brain's electrical activity during its function; recording of the brain's anatomy employing electromagnetic radiation, computer tomography (CT), and magnetic resonance imaging (MRI); and use of tracer emission-computed tomography, positron emission tomography (PET), and single-photon emission computer tomography (SPECT). Only the last methods are invasive in nature. All of these technologies provide us with a limited image of brain form and function. The story of their development spans much of the history of the convergence of modern physical and biological sciences, from the biological applications of electromagnetic radiation in the late 19th century by Roentgen to the mathematics of projection geometry by Radon early in this century, to the development of brain wave recording by Berger in the 1920s, the principles of tracer kinetics in the 1950s, and computer technology starting in the 1960s and continuing to the present day. These have given us the tools to record brain anatomy (CT and MRI) and brain function (brain evoked potentials, PET, and SPECT). There is every expectation that in each of these fields current methods will be further refined in resolution, speed, dimensionality, and sophistication of image processing.

Perhaps the future holds for us as well the development of technologies based on other physical principles or the application of electromagnetic or other radiation probes as yet unimagined that will give us new insight into how the brain functions in vivo. The superconducting quantum interference device (SQUID) is promising in this regard. For the present, let us look at each of these current technologies and pose task-specific questions.

Brain Electrical Activity Mapping

The complex process of analysis of spatial, temporal, and spectral distributions of the frequencies of brain waves produced by the electroencephalograph or the time-locked evoked potential has been considerably enhanced by the recent introduction of refined computer technology. What results is a two-dimensional image of the spatial distribution of the electrical activity of the brain for a set period following a visual, auditory, tactile, or other stimulus or complex motor act such as reading, speaking, reaching, and grasping. This allows visualization of the topographic distribution of the signals recorded through the scalp electrodes with time. The images can be displayed in rapid sequence on a color videographic video terminal, a process known as cartooning. The result is a striking image of brain electrical activity of a person listening to music, speaking, and so on. The visual system presents some very special problems for this type of recording activity because of its exposed location. For example, evoked potentials of stimuli in the right visual field destined for the left hemisphere are best recorded over the right hemisphere because of the polarity of the signal from the left. Although researchers have devised some clever methods that partially circumvent this problem, it remains an important determinant of the quality of the image from the particular brain area under study. Be that as it may, the first question we might ask is, Does the central visual field (particularly the macula) of the strabismic eye behave as does the macula of the normal eye under photopic conditions? The best stimulus to use here might be a small, haploscopically presented, briefly illuminated circular patch of sinusoidal grating with a spatial frequency of about seven cycles per second, drifting at approximately 4 hertz, as proposed by Watson and co-workers. This stimulus matches the weighting function of the most efficient photopic quantum detector in the macular region. Obviously, in the normal subject this should produce some particular pattern of electrical activity suggesting in each hemisphere a summation of the effect of the two detectors: both maculas at optimum efficiency. Stimulating each macula dichoptically should produce some fraction of the binocular potential less than the summed activity of the two maculas stimulated simultaneously (binocular summation at threshold). In the strabismic, using a haploscopic device to permit dichoptic stimulation of each macula, the same experimental paradigm should produce a normal or perhaps a *larger* than normal individual response in the macula of the fixing eye and a *smaller* than normal response when the macula of the deviated eye is stimulated (provided that eye does not take up fixation). Remember, this experiment is performed under haploscopic conditions, so that either macula (fixing or deviated) can be stimulated alone. The most plausible explanation for such a response is the effect of asynchronous activity flowing from the fixing macula to the deviated macula ("noise"). The summation of simultaneous stimulation of both maculas by this optimal detection target might very well show, because of the inherent background activity in the system, which is essentially asynchronous, the almost complete absence of any summation of potentials.

A second question that deserves to be re-asked concerns the correspondence or abnormal topographic representation of the central visual field under binocular conditions. In a small group of strabismics, McCormack demonstrated that the evoked potential response was similar when corresponding retinal points (both maculas) were stimulated and dissimilar when anomalously corresponding points were stimulated both monocularly and dichoptically. I believe that the paradigm does not, however, address the essential question, namely, how to tease out (in an inherently noisy system) the signal that represents the true abnormal connection between the macula (of the fixing eye) and the periphery (of the deviated eye). The stimulus conditions should be such that an ideal stimulus matched to the optimum weighting function of the macula of the fixing eye and the peripheral area of the nonfixing eye is employed to look at the evoked potential from both (Figure 10.1). Under these conditions, the monocular and dichoptic potentials might be predicted to exhibit similar rather than different behavior. Care in choosing and presenting the stimulus is critical if the paradigm is to be used effectively to test for the possibility of abnormal connections. Although it may be theoretically possible, I do not believe that an experiment can be run in which one locus (the macula) in the fixing eye is stimulated and a response from the periphery of the other eye is recorded; that is, the macula is stimulated in the hope of recording from the cortex representing the peripheral corresponding area of the retina in the other eye. The system is just dominated too much by the macula on an anatomic and functional basis to allow this. In summary then, brain electrical activity mapping by use of advanced computer technology should be able to answer at least two (and probably more) interesting and important questions bearing on the functional activity of the visual cortex of the strabismic as opposed to the normal subject. We must be careful, however, to make sure that the stimulus addresses the right question to the right area.

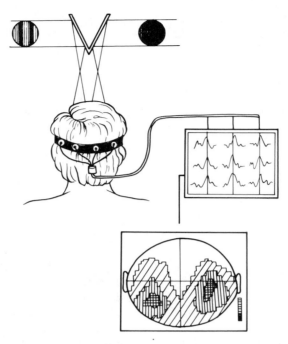

FIGURE 10.1. Haploscopic view of the optimum stimulus delivered to the left (deviated) and right eyes to examine possibly corresponding points in the binocular visual field of a strabismic subject.

Magnetic Resonance and Computer Tomography Imaging

We consider MRI and CT together because they are representatives of a single parameter requiring investigation in strabismus: the anatomy of the visual system. It is not germane to debate the merits of one or the other method of imaging, though it would seem on several grounds that MRI is the system best suited for our type of study. The appropriate questions this particular class of imagers might be expected to help answer are questions of developmental anatomy, devoid of function. The period of interest to us begins with the change in the gray/white matter ratio, which suggests a loss of water from the cortex and the beginning of myelination. This has been described by Barkovich and others in the normal human fetus and neonate. The process is not simply a deposition of myelin; rather, it comprises a change in the gray/white matter ratio accompanied by a "loss of water" in the subcortical area (Figure 10.2). This change, although not specifically further defined in the neuroradiological literature, might, in fact, be an accompaniment of the loss of subplate in the cortex (see Chapters 2 to 4) and the anatomical correlate of the "dying

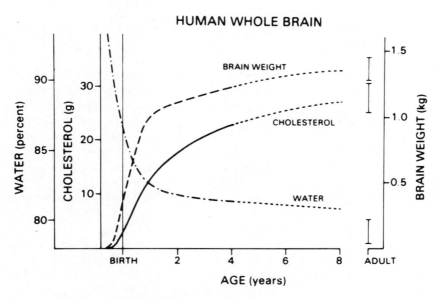

FIGURE 10.2. Changes in brain weight, water, and cholesterol with age. A precipitous drop in brain water content occurs in the perinatal period, accompanied by a rise in cholesterol content partly due to myelin. From McArdle CB, Richardson CJ, Nicholas DA, et al. Developmental features of the neonatal brain: MR Imaging. Part I: Gray-white matter differentiation and myelination. *Radiology* 1987; 162:223–229. With permission of The Radiological Society of North America.

back" of neurons, neuronal processes, and synapses in the subplate layer. This change might be a potential anatomical marker that would serve to delineate the process of absorption of subplate in the normal subject and its persistence (for an unknown period) in the strabismic. The topic is an open one on which further research in the application of this methodology is indicated. Although, on the basis of the evidence at hand, we would not be justified medically in performing imaging studies in strabismus for the sake of research alone, should careful analysis of the relevant anatomy (cortex, subplate, splenium of the corpus callosum, or other cortical or subcortical areas) demonstrate changes during development, then such studies may very well be medically indicated. At present we must use the material obtained from subjects undergoing neuroradiological imaging for other reasons. Scrutinizing this material relative to that from controls might yield clues to the anatomical changes present. Though the process is laborious, a positive finding or lack of the same in this area would be of immense importance in guiding further thinking.

Position Emission Tomography and Single-Photon Emission Computer Tomography

The imaging techniques of PET and SPECT bridge recordings of the electrical correlates of brain activity on stimulation without underlying anatomy (function without form) and with underlying anatomy of the part devoid of any correlated activity (form without function). In the proper circumstances these techniques can be used to identify connections between and within areas of the central nervous system and to map, within the brain, alterations in biochemical or physiological processes resulting from pathological or pharmacological disturbances. Indeed, preliminary PET scan results have already been reported in amblyopia, and the combined experience with PET scanning of the visual system has been well summarized by Phelps and colleagues. Whereas PET instrumentation depends for its source of imaging photons on emission of a positron by a nuclide and its annihilation by an electron, SPECT scanning depends on Technetium ^{99}m for its source of photons. Planar tomography (PET) and collimated tomography (SPECT) are employed for the formation of images. Both systems of imaging have pluses and minuses. Neither is, for every usage, the best. The clinical community is more familiar with PET scanning than with SPECT scanning. Resolution remains the single most difficult problem with both techniques. In the future, progress will probably come through improvements in image processing techniques that have been developed for processing satellite photo images.

Superconducting Quantum Interference Devices

In contrast to the devices described earlier, SQUIDs are extraordinarily sensitive to changes in the electromagnetic field and can measure such changes to the level of 10^{-14} tesla. These devices can be used to detect very faint magnetic signals associated with electrical field changes in both the heart and the brain. Magnetic field changes are not distorted by the skull as are electrical field changes. These devices have only recently appeared and remain largely research devices at this time.

Summary

The techniques described in this chapter offer us the possibility of looking at form and function together in one image. These methodologies could be adapted to the neuroradiological study of selected sites of brain metabolism in the visual system should images from brain electrical activity mapping or CT or MRI scanning provide clues as to what to look for and where to look. These high-technology imaging devices, each employing different physical principles to produce their images of form coupled with function, are not immediately adaptable to the study of strabismus. We must first formulate the appropriate question from a knowledge of form and function gathered elsewhere. Nevertheless, we do well to review what is available in this dynamic field for I believe different versions of these techniques will be used diagnostically in the field of strabismus.

This chapter has offered but a brief overview of special types of advanced imaging technology that perhaps will pay dividends in our study of strabismus. We must carefully organize the search, employ test stimuli designed to maximize the signal from tissues of the visual system, and process those signals with the best image enhancers to obtain maximum resolution. A conceivable goal would be an organized program of research employing the noninvasive technology primarily to discover clues, anatomical and/or functional, and the more invasive technology to fit form and function together. To bring these to focus on our problem would be, in a sense, to achieve at least part of Goethe's dream of science: the study of objects and phenomena in their natural habitat.

11
What Can We Learn from Developmental Neuropathology?

Since the full grown forest turns out to be impenetrable and indefinable, why not revert to the study of young wood in the nursery stage, as we might say.

Santiago Ramon y Cajal

With this chapter, I hope to invite the interested reader with the special talents of the neuropathologist and a sense of curiosity to follow a pathway seldom trod—the systematic investigation in donor material of aspects of the developing visual system that might further elucidate the anatomical nature of the lesion in strabismus. Although a singular path, I can point to at least one contemporary area of study of this sort that has added greatly to our knowledge of a problem in some respects not unlike strabismus. Dyslexia has probably been with us since language above a grunt emerged in the human, though it has not been recognized as such. Spoken language has been in existence on the order of 100,000 years; written language, limited to a few scholars at first who were self selected *for* facility with spoken and written language and *against* dyslexia for perhaps 10,000 years. Reading and writing skills were not acquired by the majority of the population until the printing press and mass public education and have probably been in existence for several hundred years at most. The medical definition of dyslexia was not formulated until the late 19th/early 20th century by Pringle-Morgan and Hinshelwood; the latter defined it as "congenital word blindness" because of its similarity to acquired "wort blindheit" contemporaneously described by Kussmaul. Hinshelwood, a Scottish ophthalmologist, speculated that a lesion in the language area of the brain recently described by Paul Broca might account for the syndrome. There the matter lay for more than half a century while dyslexia literally became a pedagogical "football"; theories, speculations, and abstractions by educators, psychologists, psychiatrists, neurologists, child developmentalists, and other interested parties accumulated until somebody had the good sense to look at anatomy first in the normal person and then in the abnormal person. Although the rest is not yet history, the size equality of the planum temporale in the right and left hemispheres in 17 consecutive autopsied dyslexics, as opposed to a 20% to 40% size difference between right to left planam in the normal person, is a very important anatomical finding regardless of how it came about. The point is that until the 1970s, no one had taken the trouble to look at the anatomy, as first suggested by Hinshelwood.

I use this story to illustrate my point: "We do not know until we look." Today we have the tools that skilled personnel need to perform axoplasmic flow studies on postmortem material. Other modern methods, including modifications of Golgi methods, intracellular injection of dyes and enzymes (horseradish peroxidase and others), autoradiography using tracer amino acids, electron microscopy, and immunocytochemistry, have enabled us to characterize in part the parameters of growth and development as well as the synaptology of the central nervous system. For example, the labeling of cortical cells with retrograde axoplasmic tracers has conclusively demonstrated that only pyramidal cells are the major output cells of the cortex. The input to these cells has also been characterized. [^{3}H]Thymidine autoradiography as used by Rakic, Jones, and co-workers has enabled us to begin to understand the ontogenesis of the cortex from neuronal birth through migration to the formation of the cortical plate (see Chapter 2 for a review).

On the other hand, through studies of regional blood flow and metabolism and histochemical detection of oxidative and metabolic cells (particularly cytochrome oxidase–rich cells) our understanding of structure has been coupled with function.

Each of the preceding chapters has defined part of an "in vivo" research program to uncover evidence that strabismus too has a predictable pattern of defects most parsimoniously explained by positing a central nervous system malformation as an etiology. Chapter 10 showed how this can be brought closer to realization by using modern imaging technology to focus on the visual brain. The final step then is to turn to the anatomy and look for the anatomical form that might provide a substrate for disturbance of function. In this context, our task is to define in broad terms an anatomical site for neuropathological investigation. The goal of such research would be to comprehend the interrelationships among the various components of the primitive marginal layer of the visual cortex and its overall organization. Let us start with some idea of how this layer is established. The first step is arrival of corticopetal fibers at the undifferentiated telencephalic vesicle early in embryonic development (probably about the 50th day in humans). These fibers form within the telencephalic vesicle a superficial or external white matter layer called the marginal layer or zone. Primitive neurons in this layer establish a fibrilloneuronal organization called the primordial plexiform layer. Although of short duration, this layer is functionally active, as primitive synaptic vesicles and contacts have been demonstrated between its fibers and neurons. This is the first time and site worth investigating in the search for a pathoanatomical basis for strabismus.

A short time later the second major transformation in cortical ontogenesis takes place, the appearance of the cortical plate, devoid of neurons, separating the primitive marginal layer into two cell-rich layers, a mantle and a subplate layer, with the cell-free cortical plate between. This cell-free zone is the future neo-cortex. Migrating neuroblasts destined to form the mature cortex accumulate in the subplate layer. Neurons segregated into the mantle layer are differentiated into horizontal cells, called Cajal-Retzius neurons. All pyramidal neurons, when they later invade the future cortical plate, anchor their apical dendritic bouquet on the cell processes of these Cajal-Retzius neurons. The subplate layer, as noted previously, is a rich neuropil with neurons and synapses destined to disappear. This second step in cortical ontogenesis—the division of the primitive marginal layer into mantle and subplate, both synaptically active—may provide a site and time for neuropathological investigation. It is this early cortical organization stage characterized by functionally active synapses above and below but not in the cortical plate itself that might play a key role in determining the final form and function of the cortical connections to come. Perhaps minor or major abnormalities in these key primitive layers produce the lesion that leads to strabismus. Certainly, their role in providing the scaffold necessary for the "inside out" organization of cortical pyramids has been well documented, suggesting a key role in the later morphogenesis of the adult cortex. Well before the cortical pyramids receive any other afferent input, such as specific and nonspecific thalamic afferents and callosal and other intracortical fibers, there is evidence that these primitive neuronal networks are forming aminergic, functionally active synapses very early in development.

Cortical development during this period might furnish important anatomical clues to the ontogenesis of strabismus. Once again, an area of primitive development holds our interest. This primitive development is part of a normal nervous system developmental process which, as newer cortical structures develop around it, undergoes normal degeneration and disappears. The goal of anatomical studies would be to see if the primitive persists beyond its useful life or undergoes another, unknown transformation. A disorder of this primitive network might be just what the father of all neurodevelopmental studies, Ramon y Cajal, had in mind when he wrote the words with which this chapter began.

12
What of the Future?

We err if we expect more enlightenment from a hypothesis than from the facts themselves.

Ernst Mach

In closing this book I feel that I have completed a journey, with my readers as companions. The words of Ernst Mach, the great natural scientist, biophysicist (before the word was coined), and philosopher of the turn of the century are apt ones to keep before us at all times. The primary purpose of this book was to ask questions: questions I deemed important in deepening and broadening our knowledge of strabismus; questions that seem to be within our collective power as a community of basic and clinical scientists and practitioners to answer; questions that because of their factual answers, will lead to progress in the study of strabismus akin to the progress being made elsewhere in our specialty; questions, the answers to which may provide insight into both form and function of the visual nervous system, of interest to psychophysical, developmental, and neurobiological colleagues as well as ourselves.

In each of the preceding chapters, I have reflected on and summarized, to the extent possible, the body of knowledge current within the various disciplines; most of this knowledge was not my own, but directly bears on our central topic. It should be clear that I am no expert in these fields, but rather an interested bystander. Because of that interest, I have posed questions within the framework of these separate disciplines that may shed light on some aspect of our topic. These questions, all of which derive from the central anatomical hypothesis of the nature of strabismus, constitute the core of a research program within and across these disciplines. In each I have endeavored to ask what seemed to me the best, most central and telling questions. In so doing, I am attempting to engage many other (and brighter) minds to apply the tools of their discipline to our subject. I am not issuing a harsh challenge but rather extending a warm hand of welcome to begin a journey to "knowledge to come," which is bound to be full of surprises, delights, mysteries, paradoxes, and insights central to our grasp of how the nervous system is put together and works. What a delightful vista the next decade and beyond, the 21st century, presents us!

Let us put our problem in several contexts to better grasp it. In its simplest conception, strabismus is the result of an atavistic persistence of a structure that plays a central role in the development of the visual nervous system: Synaptic connections in the subplate layer of the cortex are destined to disappear along with that layer later in development. When they do not disappear, strabismus results. That is the essence of our hypothesis. In other contexts, clinicians are quite familiar with structures that arise and flourish during development of the visual system, only to undergo decline, cell death, and removal during later development. The tunica vasculosa lentis, the primary vitreous, and the optic stalk are but a few familiar examples. Each has a clinical phenomenology associated with the persistence of the embryological structure beyond its useful life. So in this sense might we conceive of strabismus.

On a deeper level, the problem raised by the intricate pattern of development and maldevelopment of form and function of the visual system is best understood in its most elemental terms as a topobiological problem. Topobiology, a term coined by Gerald Edelman, is the study of site-dependent interactions at the surface of living cells that regulate processes of embryological development. It encompasses both the driving forces of cell division, migration, and death and the regulatory processes, particularly cell adhesion (synapse formation). It is on this level that the problem of strabismus has its most profound meaning. Undoubtedly, both the genetic code and epigenetic forces have central roles in the development and maldevelopment of the visual system. Thus the basic tools and concepts of molecular biology must be used to probe the nature of strabismus.

I began this journey with a troubled spirit—a sense that so much in my special area of interest, strabismus, had remained unchanged, as if asleep, in the quarter of a century I have been a physician and ophthalmologist. On a deeper level, I realized that although almost nothing done today to treat cataracts, glaucoma, and retinal detachment is the same as it was 25 years ago. To treat strabismus I was using a patch almost three centuries old, an operation one and one-half centuries old and spectacles, which were introduced a century ago. Writing this book has for me been what the Greeks aptly named catharsis, a cleansing and purification, and a journey, a period of travel and growth. One has but to pause for a moment to reflect on and be filled with a sense of wonder at the beauty of the central nervous system. From simple building blocks and processes, an immense, complex, powerful cathedral is built. On contemplation of the putative extent of the lesion (regardless of its site, timing, and process) giving rise to strabismus, one cannot help but be astonished at how much is preserved as normal in spite of the lesion.

The story of the development of the nervous system, told in this book schematically, is and must remain one of the marvels of all biology, probably second only to life itself in its interest to us. It is not without irony and yet at the same time fortuitous that so many disciplines, each with a different perspective (neuroembryology, neural network theory, artificial intelligence, visual psychophysics, molecular genetics, medical genetics, teratology, developmental medicine, pediatric neurology, neuroradiology, and opthalmology), will influence study of the clinical problem that is the subject of this book. I believe that strabismus has not excited the same interest in the discipline of ophthalmology in the past decades as have intraocular lenses, refractive surgery, and lasers simply because we have had to wait for other sciences to mature and provide the handles with which we can grasp our problem. It is up to us to continue and move forward in every field possible. And although one cannot dictate the course of research any more than one can control human thought, the greatest goal this book could achieve is to induce knowledgeable people in the various disciplines to examine every tenet of the central hypothesis and its derivative predictions carefully. If, as a result, the hypothesis is proved wrong, without doubt, other, more fertile hypotheses will emerge on which to build our science. In so doing, this book will have challenged all of us to think seriously and deeply about strabismus in its many and varied manifestations. We can do no less than that for the beautiful children who have it.

Bibliography

Introduction

This book is speculative in nature, and obviously I cannot give citations for ideas and hypotheses yet to be tested! What I have attempted to do instead is give the reader a flavor of the references I consulted in the generation of each chapter. I make no claim for their being exhaustive on any of the chapters; rather, they proved fruitful in the germination of ideas set forth. Many of the references are obviously not in my discipline. To guard against the possibility of an egregious error on my part, I have, in addition to reading the references as carefully as possible, consulted with experts in the various disciplines, in many cases the authors themselves, to ensure my interpretation was not off the mark. Often, the cited reference has no apparent direct connection to the text. I ask the reader's forbearance because the work cited deepened and broadened my knowledge of the central nervous system, particularly the stage of early development. It is here in this organ and at this stage that I believe the genesis of the condition strabismus lies. The references may then have opened for me a new way of conceiving of the function of part of the nervous system and thus helped to extend and expand the ways in which I came to look at the subject of this book.

On still another level, notes and references might be misleading, invidious, and inadequate. Misleading because most of the material in this book is not based on a single source or combination of sources. Rather, the material represents my own thoughts cued by reading many sources. Citing only a few references would not have reflected the process. Moreover, to leave out any major work while citing others would be invidious, an injustice to the authors not cited. In short, a traditional reference list would have been inadequate for specialists and of no use to nonspecialists. Note, however, that the first citation for each chapter is the source of that chapter's opening quotation. Finally, one pleasure in putting this book together has been the opportunity, unparalleled in my life's experience, to think deeply and speculate about the true nature of strabismus — to delve beyond its phenomenology and use my mind and my imagination to visualize what the brain of the child with strabismus might look like. I would be less than candid with the reader if I did not confess that this is the real joy in writing this book.

The references noted for each chapter then are simple guideposts directing my journey. I would not want the reader to hold any of the innocent and careful authors of the books, monographs, and articles cited responsible for my speculations, which some may judge inept or perhaps label "flights of fancy." With these simple cautions in mind, let us then together look at where my journey started for each chapter.

Preface

Rothman KJ. Causes. *Am J Epidemiol* 1976;104:587–592. This article is the single best exposition of the notion of causality as the word is employed today in science and medicine. Though it takes several readings to grasp the meaning of the author's carefully chosen words, it is well worth the effort to the reader.

Goethe JW, in a letter to Frau von Stein as quoted by Magnus R. *Goethe as a Scientist*. Translated by H. Norden. New York: H. Shuman; 1949:43. Goethe was profoundly concerned with the increasing abstraction he noted in the developing sciences of his time. He rebelled against it and felt that we must learn about nature by studying the phenomena of nature in their (natural) environment. The world of science passed him by, yet his concerns were real and important, as witness the comments of Werner Heisenberg on Goethe's approach to science in *Traditions in Science*. New York: Seabury Press; 1983:12, 130.

Chapter 1

Ross WD, ed. *Aristotle's Metaphysics*. Oxford: Clarendon Press; 1924: Vol. 1, Book 2, Chap. 1, B993A3–B24.

Reed C. *Hilbert, by Constance Reed*. New York/Heidelberg/Berlin: Springer-Verlag; 1970:1–244. Of the many contributions Hilbert made to mathematics, his 1900 lecture stands out as a masterpiece. Most of us are familiar with Goedel's theorem which disproved one of Hilbert's most cherished hypotheses, namely, that mathematics was internally consistent and logical and could be derived from first principles. His questions are still with us today and serve as a fertile source of work for young mathematicians. The lecture itself was printed as "Mathematische Probleme" in *Ann Phys Math* 1900:44–63, 213–237.

Isaac Newton, *General Scholium of Principia Mathematica*, 1713, as cited by Jacobson M. *Developmental Neurobiology*. New York: Plenum Press; 1978:344. In Newton's time hypotheses abounded, and alchemy was considered as real as the infant science of chemistry. Newton's dictum opposed the idle generation of hypotheses that could not be tested.

Westheimer G. In: Lennerstrand G, von Noorden GK, Campos EC, eds. *Strabismus and Amblyopia*. New York: Plenum Press; 1988: Chap. 33, 413–416. Gerald Westheimer is right in carefully separating hypotheses in the physical sciences with their rigor and mathematical formalism as opposed to those in the biological sciences. He is also correct, I believe, in stating that strabismus does not have a theory worthy of the name. But see also in this regard, Crick FW, *What Mad Pursuit*, New York: Basic Books; 1988: Chap. 10, 108–115, on the limits of biological hypotheses and the inherent variability of all outcomes of biological experiments, even when they are done correctly, as by physicists such as Crick!

Popper K. As cited by Heisenberg W. *Traditions in Science*. New York: Seabury Press; 1983:125. Popper, the philosopher of science, has neatly placed limits on the value of any scientific hypothesis—it's only as good as its last affirmation.

Medawar PD. *Induction and Intuition in Scientific Thought*. Philadelphia: American Philosophical Society; 1969. It is useful to read this deeply insightful work in conjunction with Heisenberg's work cited earlier.

Von Monakaw K. As cited by Pasik P, Pasik T. In: Bender M, ed. *Oculomotor System*. New York: Hoeber Medical Division, Harper & Row; 1961:63. Von Monakaw's statement is perhaps more true and has more anatomical bases than when he made it. Such is the function of the intuition of genius.

Chapter 2

von Neuman J. The general and logical theory of automata. In: Jeffress LA, ed. *Cerebral Mechanisms in Behavior*. New York/London: Hafner; 1951:1–41.

Sidman RL, Rakic P. Development of the human central nervous system. In: Haymaker W, Adams RD, eds. *Histology and Histopathology of the Nervous System*. Springfield, Ill: CC Thomas; 1982:3–145. This chapter served very much as a model for the preparation of Chapter 2. Its bibliography (which I consulted liberally) is encyclopedic and served as the framework for all that followed on the ontogenesis of the nervous system. I am indebted to Pasco Rakic for many helpful comments and criticisms as well as for his profound insights into central nervous system development.

Moore KL. *The Developing Human: Clinically Oriented Embryology*. 3rd ed. Philadelphia: WB Saunders; 1988. This clinically oriented text is very lucid, particularly on the vulnerability of the eyes and central nervous system in sharing common responses to the actions of teratogens. It is from this text that the idea of strabismus as a dysmorphology began to germinate.

Jacobson M. *Developmental Neurobiology*. 2nd ed. New York: Plenum Press; 1978. This was my second most frequently consulted source text for the materials and concepts developed in this chapter. It looks at the processes involved in neurogenesis from a different angle than do Sidman and Rakic. The views provided by the two are complementary not contradictory.

Menkes JH. *Textbook of Child Neurology*. 3rd ed. Philadelphia: Lea & Febiger; 1985. Also quite informative in the area of the linkage between time and developmental anatomy.

O'Rahilly R, Gardner E: The timing and sequence of events in the development of the human nervous system during the embryonic period proper. *Z Anat Entwicklungsgesch* 1971;134:1–12. This work made clear, when I read the original, the complex interplay between spatial foldings and flexures that moves the process of development from a simple straight neural tube to the beginnings of a recognizable brain.

Anatomy of the Nervous System

Rather than cite a single reference, I cite together the modern textbooks of neuroanatomy that I consulted freely for further elaboration and understanding of the form of the adult central nervous system:

Carpenter MB, Sutin J, eds. *Human Neuroanatomy.* 8th ed. Baltimore: Williams & Wilkins; 1983.

Ranson SW. *The Anatomy of the Nervous System.* 10th ed. revised by Clark SL. Philadelphia: WB Saunders; 1959.

Truex RC, Carpenter MB: *Strong and Elwyn's Human Neuroanatomy.* 6th ed. Baltimore: Williams and Wilkins; 1969.

Wolstenholme GEW, O'Connor M, eds. *Growth of the Nervous System: A Ciba Foundation Symposium.* Boston: Little, Brown; 1968.

Early Neurogenesis

Yokoh Y. The early development of the nervous system in man. *Acta Anat* 1968;71: 492–518.

Fujita S. Kinetics of cellular proliferation. *Exp Cell Res* 1962;28:52–60.

These two are excellent descriptions of the process of early neurogenesis.

Rakic P. DNA synthesis and cell division in the adult primate brain. *Ann NY Acad Sci* 1985;457:193–211.

Rakic P. Limits of neurogenesis in primates. *Science* 1985;227:1054–1056.

These two complete the picture.

Peters A, Palay SL, Webster deF. *The Fine Structure of The Nervous System: The Neurones and Supporting Cells.* Philadelphia: WB Saunders; 1976:232–233. A concise and clear account of the electron microscopic picture of the interplay between neurons and glia.

Migration and Synaptogenesis

Rakic P. Specification of cerebral cortical areas. *Science* 1988;241:170–176. This is a seminal account of the process by which neurons, once born, migrate to their destiny in the cortex.

Easter SS, Purves D, Rakic P, Spitzer NC. The changing view of neural specificity. *Science* 1985;230:507–511. This article presents the modern view of the limits and possibilities of neuronal specificity. It seems to depart somewhat from the older rigid formalism of the neuronal doctrine.

Morest DK. The growth of dendrites in the mammalian brain. *Z Anat Entwicklungsgesch* 1969;128:290–317. A thorough anatomical and morphological treatment of the process of synaptogenesis as it occurs in mammalian brain. It cannot be very different in a human.

Rakic P. Prenatal development of the visual system in rhesus monkey. *Philos Trans R Soc London [Biol]* 1977;278:245–260. A superb report of the ontogenesis of the primate monkey visual nervous system using pulse-labeled tracer methodology, a technique pioneered by the author that promises to shed more light on central nervous system development as its use is expanded, particularly in collaboration with the other radiochemical, histochemical, and enzymatic and molecular genetic probes available today.

Rakic P. Guidance of neurons migrating to the fetal monkey neocortex. *Brain Res* 1971;33:471–476.

Rakic P. Mode of cell migration to the superficial layers of fetal monkey neocortex. *J Comp Neurol* 1972;145:61–83.

These two articles describe clearly what must happen to neurons on their journey from birth to their penetration of the otherwise empty cortical plate to begin the process of formation of the fetal cortex.

Myelination

Yakovlev PI, Lecours AR. The myelogenetic cycles of regional maturation of the brain. In: Minkowski A, ed. *Regional Development of the Brain in Early Life*. Oxford: Blackwell Scientific; 1967:3–70. This is the classic account of the process of myelinate as seen to occur in the human collection of the late Dr. Yakovlev. It is the definitive work on this topic up to the date of its publication.
Richardson EP Jr. Myelination in the human central nervous system. In: Haymaker W, Adams RD, eds. *Histology and Histopathology of the Nervous System*. Springfield, Ill: CC Thomas; 1982:Chap. 2, 146–173.

Neural Networks (Organization and Form) Leading to Their Function)

Edelman GM. Group selection and phasic reentrant signaling: A theory of higher brain function. In: Schmitt FO, Worden FG, eds. *The Neurosciences, Fourth Study Program*. Cambridge, MA: MIT Press; 1978:1115–1139.
Cowan WM. Selection and control in neurogenesis. Ibid:59–79.
Singer W. Central-core control of visual-cortex functions. Ibid:1093–1110.
Van Essen DC, Maunsell JHR. Hierarchical organization and functional streams in the visual cortex. *Trends Neurosci* 1983;6:370–374.

These sources gave me insight into the nervous system as an epithelial tissue, its similarity to other epithelia and to the immune system, its various feedback and feedforward loops that modulate and control its function. These and other contributions from these MIT study programs proved helpful in germinating the ideas put forward in this book.

Histogenesis Within the Visual Nervous System

Hendrickson A, Rakic P. Histogenesis and synaptogenesis in the dorsal lateral geniculate nucleus (LGd) of the fetal monkey brain. *Anat Rec* 1977;187:602.
LeVay S, Connolly M, Houde J, Van Essen DC. The complete pattern of ocular dominance stripes in the striate cortex and visual field of the macaque monkey. *J Neurosci* 1985;5:486–501.
Nelson SB, LeVay S. Topographic organization of the optic radiation of the cat. *J Comp Neurol* 1985;240:322–330.
Voigt T, LeVay S, Stamnes MA. Morphological and immunocytochemical observations on the visual callosal projections in the cat. *J Comp Neurol* 1988;272:450–460.

I have borrowed from works such as these many of my ideas on when, where, and how the human central nervous system forms. The process in cats and monkeys probably comes closest to resembling what happens in our species and this probably is as close as we are going to come in describing the process. The last article is the best description I have read of the developing geometry of the cortical ocular dominance stripes in the monkey and its dependence on afferent input by thalamocortical radiation.

Development of the Human and Primate Fovea and Retina

Curcio CA, Sloan KR Jr, Packer O, Hendrickson AE, Kalina RE. Distribution of cones in human and monkey retina: Individual variability and radial asymmetry. *Science* 1987; 236:579–582.

Yuodelis C, Hendrickson AE. A qualitative and quantitative analysis of the human fovea during development. *Vision Res* 1986;26:847–855.

Hendrickson AE, Youdalis C. The morphological development of the human fovea. *Ophthalmology* 1984;91:603–612.

These three works coupled with Nishimura and Rakic's works (following) on retinal ontogenesis in the monkey provide the best insight available to the histogenesis of the retina.

Nishimura Y, Rakic P. Development of the rhesus monkey retina. II. A three-dimensional analysis of the sequences of synaptic combinations in the inner plexiform layer. *J Comp Neurol* 1987;262:290–313.

Nishimura Y, Rakic P. Synaptogenesis in the primate retina proceeds from the ganglion cells towards the photoreceptors. *Neurosci Res Suppl* 1987;6:S253–S268.

Disorders of Neuronal Migration, Ectopias

Rakic P. Cell migration and neuronal ectopias in the brain. *Birth Defects* 1975;11(7): 95–129. In this article, Rakic details failure of migration giving rise to ectopias and heterotopias associated with a number of diverse clinical syndromes such as trisomy 18, lissencephaly, and ataxia telangiectasia. Clearly, the type of disease associated with migration defects does not conform to our clinical topic of interest, strabismus.

Corpus Callosum, Its Anatomy and Function

Berlucchi G. Anatomical and physiological aspects of visual functions of the corpus callosum. *Brain Res* 1972;37:371–392.

Elberger AJ. The functional role of the corpus callosum in the developing visual systems: A review. *Prog Neurobiol* 1982;18:15–79.

Innocenti GM. General organization of callosal connections in the cerebral cortex. In: Jones EG, Peters A, eds. *Cerebral Cortex.* Vol. 5: *Sensory-Motor Areas and Aspects of Cortical Connectivity.* New York: Plenum Press; 1986:291–353.

Clearly, the corpus callosum is of interest to us with respect to potential anatomical study and verification of the central hypothesis of this book. These three references set out in great detail (with appropriate bibliographies) what we know of the structure and its importance to vision, particularly binocular vision and its function. In addition, see the work of Voigt, LeVay, and Stamnes already cited.

Detailed Anatomy of Various Animal Models of Miswiring

Guillery RW. An abnormal retinogeniculate projection in Siamese cats. *Brain Res* 1969;14:1739–1741.

Hubel DH, Wiesel TN. Aberrant visual projections in the Siamese cat. J Physiol 1971;218:33–62.

Kliot M, Shatz CJ. Abnormal development of the retinogeniculate projection in Siamese cats. *J Neurosci* 1985;5:2641–2653.

Shatz CJ. Anatomy of interhemispheric connections in the visual system of Boston Siamese and ordinary cats. *J Comp Neurol* 1977;173:497–518.

Shatz C. A comparison of the visual pathways in Boston and Midwestern Siamese cats. *J Comp Neurol* 1977;171:205–228.

Shatz C. Abnormal interhemispheric connections in the visual system of Boston Siamese cats: A physiological study. *J Comp Neurol* 1977;171:229–245.

Shatz CJ. Anatomy of interhemispheric connections of the visual system of Boston Siamese and ordinary cats. *J Comp Neurol* 1977;173:497–518.

Shatz CJ, Kliot M. Prenatal misrouting of the retinogeniculate pathway in Siamese cats. *Nature* 1982;300:525–529.

Shatz CJ, LeVay S. Siamese cat: Altered connections of the visual cortex. *Science* 1979;204:328–330.

Webster MJ, Shatz CJ, Kliot M, Silver J. Abnormal pigmentation and unusual morphogenesis of the optic stalk may be correlated with retinal axon misguidance in embryonic Siamese cats. *J Comp Neurol* 1988;269:592–611.

These works clearly summarize what is known about the abnormalities of wiring in the afferent visual system that give rise to the defects in Siamese cats. These result from abnormal operation of the albino gene controlling neuronal migration, which differs from its abnormal operation with respect to pigment and epithelial tissues.

Synaptogenesis

Bourgeois JP, Jastreboff PJ, Rakic P. Synaptogenesis in the visual cortex of normal and preterm monkeys: Evidence of intrinsic regulation of synaptic overproduction. *Proc Natl Acad Sci USA* 1989;86:4297–4301.

Cooper ML, Rakic P. Gradients of cellular maturation and synaptogenesis in superior colliculus of the fetal rhesus monkey. *J Comp Neurol* 1983;215:165–186.

Huttenlocher PR, De Courten C, Garey LJ, Van der Loos H. Synaptogenesis in human visual cortex—Evidence for synapse elimination during normal development. *Neurosci Lett* 1982;33:247–252.

Rakic P, Bourgeois JP, Eckenhoff MF, Zecevic N, Goldman-Rakic PS. Concurrent overproduction of synapses in diverse regions of the primate cerebral cortex. *Science* 1986;232:232–235.

Williams RW, Rakic P. Elimination of neurons from the rhesus monkey's lateral geniculate nucleus during development. *J Comp Neurol* 1988;272:424–436.

These articles summarize the state of our knowledge of the process of synaptogenesis within the central nervous system. Much of what is to follow in this book is concerned, to a greater or lesser extent, with this process. These papers then are seminal, concerned as they are with the parameters, the kinetics, the influence brought to bear, and the modulation of the process of synaptogenesis.

Subplate

Chun JJM, Shatz CJ. Redistribution of synaptic vesicle antigen is correlated with the dis-appearance of a transient synaptic zone in the developing cerebral cortex. *Neuron* 1988;1:297–310.

Chun JJM, Nakamura MJ, Shatz CJ. Transient cells of the developing mammalian telen-cephalon are peptide-immunoreactive neurons. *Nature* 1987;325:617–620.

Chun JJM, Schatz CJ. A fibronectin-like molecule is present in the developing cat cerebral cortex and is correlated with subplate neurons. *J Cell Biol* 1988;106:857–872.

Kostovic I, Rakic P: Cytology and time of origin of interstitial neurons in the white matter in infant and adult human and monkey telencelphalon. *J Neurocytol* 1980;9:219–242.

Rakic P. Limits of neurogenesis in primates. *Science* 1985;227:1054–1055.

Shatz CJ, Chun JJM, Luskin MB. The role of subplate in the developing mammalian telen-cephalon. In Peters A, Jones EG, eds. *Cerebral Cortex*. Vol. 7: *Development and Matu-ration of Cerebral Cortex*. New York: Plenum Press; 1988:35–58.

These references are of central importance to the rest of this book. They detail what is known about subplate, which is destined to arise, flourish, degenerate, dis-appear, and be replaced by white matter in the cerebral cortex. The references make clear that it is not some chimeric structure, but must play an integral role in the genesis of the future cortical plate. It is the most likely candidate for the persis-tence of a structure that might give rise to strabismus.

Neuronal Death and Normal Development

Gage FH, Bjorklund A. Trophic and growth regulating mechanisms in the central nervous system monitored by intracerebral neural transplants. *Ciba Found Symp* 1987;126:143–159.

O'Leary DDM. Remodelling of early axonal projections through the selective elimination of neurons and long axon collaterals. *Ciba Found Symp* 1987;126:113–142.

Thoenen H, Barde YA, Davies AM, Johnson JE. Neurotrophic factors and neuronal death. *Ciba Found Symp* 1987;126:82–95.

Hormonal Control of Neuronal Death in Invertebrates

Truman JW, Schwartz LM. Steroid regulation of neuronal death in the moth nervous sys-tem. *J Neurosci* 1984;4:274–280.

Hormonal Control of Neuronal Death in the Amphibian

Kimmel CB, Model P: Developmental studies of the Mauthner cell. In: Faber DS, Korn H, eds. *Neurobiology of the Mauthner Cell*. New York: Raven Press; 1978:183–220.

Hormonal Control of Neuronal Death in the Rat

Breedlove SM, Jordan CL, Arnold AP. Neurogenesis of motor neurons in the sexually dimorphic spinal nucleus of the bulbocavernosus in rats. *Brain Res* 1983;285:39–43.

Chapter 3

Opitz JM, Herrmann J, Pettersen JC, Bersu ET, Colacino SC. Terminological, diagnostic, nosological and anatomical-developmental aspects of developmental defects in man. *Adv Hum Genet* 1979;9:71–164.

Teratology

Holmes LB, et al. *Mental Retardation: An Atlas of Diseases with Associated Physical Abnormalities*. New York: MacMillan; 1972.

Miller RW. The discovery of human teratogens, carcinogens and mutagens: Lessons for the future. *Chem Mutag* 1976;5:101–126.

Schardein JL. *Chemically Induced Birth Defects*. New York: Marcel Dekker; 1985.

Sever JL, Brent RL, eds. *Teratogen Update. Environmentally Induced Birth Defect Risks*. New York: Alan R. Liss; 1986.

Shepard TH. *Catalog of Teratogenic Agents*. 3rd ed. Baltimore: Johns Hopkins University Press; 1980.

Wilson JG. Environmental factors: Teratogenic drugs. In: Brent RL, Harris MI, eds. *Prevention of Embryonic, Fetal, and Perinatal Disease*. DHEW 76-853 (NIH). Washington, DC: U.S. Government Printing Office; 1976:147–161.

Wilson JG, Fraser FC, eds. *Handbook of Teratology*. New York: Plenum Press; 1977:Vol. 1–3.

Warkany J. The susceptibility of the fetus and child to chemical pollutants. Problems in applying teratologic observations in animals to man. *Pediatrics* 1974;53:820.

These various works that I consulted in eclectic fashion furnished me with an insight into how potent and devastating the wrong substance at the wrong time can be to the developing embryo and fetus.

The Operation of Genes

Lemire RJ, Loesser JD, et al. *Normal and Abnormal Development of the Human Nervous System*. Hagerstown, Md: Harper & Row, 1975.

McKusick VA. *Mendelian Inheritance in Man: Catalogues of Autosomal Dominant, Autosomal Recessive, and X-Linked Phenotypes*. 5th ed. Baltimore: Johns Hopkins University Press; 1978.

Both of these books provided me with insight into how genes operate.

Strabismus as It Relates to this Particular Chapter

Chavasse FB. *Worth's Squint* or *The Binocular Reflexes and the Treatment of Strabismus*. 7th ed. Philadelphia: P. Blackiston's Son; 1939.

Donders FC. Zur Pathogenie des Schielens. *Albrecht von Graefes Arch Ophthalmol* 1863;9:99–154.

Duane A. A new classification of the motor anomalies of the eyes based upon physiological principles. *Ann Ophthalmol* 1896;4:969. 1897;6:84, 247.

Ebers Papyrus (circa 1500 BC). Cited in Duke Elder S, ed. *System of Ophthalmology*. Vol. 6: *Ocular Motility and Strabismus*. St. Louis: CV Mosby; 1973:223.

Keiner GBJ. *New Viewpoints on the Origin of Squint: A Clinical and Statistical Study on Its Nature, Cause and Therapy*. The Hague: Martinus Nijhoff; 1951.

Parinaud H. Rapport sur le traitement du strabisme. *Bull Mem Soc Fr Ophthalmol* 1893;11:93–196.

Von Graefe A. Beitrage zur Physiologie und Pathologie der schiefen Augenmuskeln. *Albrecht von Graefes Arch Ophthalmol* 1854;1:1–82.

Worth C. *Squint: Its Causes, Pathology and Treatment*. 4th ed. London: John Bale and Danielson; 1915.

I found it illuminating to consult the original works of the masters. These are the original references in these areas with the exception of *Ebers Papyrus*, which is cited from another source.

Chapter 4

Aristotle. *On Man in the Universe*, edited by Loomis LR. Roslyn, NY: W.J. Blank Inc.; 1943:Book 1, Chap. 2, 248.

This chapter is the keystone in the arch of this book. All that preceded it has led to this point and all that follows is derivative of it in some fashion. It contains, in addition to the formal statement of my hypothesis on the nature of strabismus, a description of the generic model of strabismus to which the hypothesis applies. Obviously, all that I have read and experienced as a clinician bears on it for such background material. I remain grateful to the authors of the standard textbooks on strabismus.

Crone RA. *Diplopia*. Amsterdam: Excerpta Medica; 1973.

Duke Elder S, Wybar K. *System of Ophthalmology*. Vol. VI: *Ocular Motility and Strabismus*. St. Louis: CV Mosby; 1973.

Hugonnier R, Clayette-Hugonnier S. *Strabismus, Heterophoria, and Ocular Motor Paralysis: Clinical Ocular Muscle Imbalance*. Translated by Veronneau-Troutman S. St. Louis: CV Mosby; 1969.

Lennerstrand G, Zee DS, Keller EL, eds. *Functional Basis of Ocular Motility Disorders: Proceedings of a Wenner-Gren Center and Smith-Kettlewell Eye Research Foundation International Symposium, held in Wenner-Gren Center, Stockholm, 31 August–3 September 1981*. Oxford/New York: Pergamon Press; 1982.

Lyle TK, Bridgeman GJO. *Worth and Chavasse's Squint: The Binocular Reflexes and the Treatment of Strabismus*. 9th ed. London: Bailliere, Tindall and Cox; 1959.

Ogle KN, Martens TG, Dyer JA. *Ocular Motor Imbalance in Binocular Vision and Fixation Disparity*. Philadelphia: Lea & Febiger; 1967.

Parks MM, Mitchell PR, Wheeler MB, eds. *Ocular Motility and Strabismus*. Volume 1 in: Tasman W, Jaeger EA, eds. *Duane's Clinical Ophthalmology*. Philadelphia: JB Lippincott; 1989.

Reinecke RD, Parks MM. *Strabismus: A Programmed Text*. 3rd ed. Norwalk, Conn: Appleton & Lange; 1987. *Strabismis Ophthalmic Symposia: Proceedings of the New Orleans Academy of Ophthalmology*. St. Louis: CV Mosby; 1950, 1956, 1961, 1970, 1977.

Scobee RG. *The Ocular Rotary Muscles*. 2nd ed. St. Louis: CV Mosby; 1952.

Von Noorden GK. *Binocular Vision Monocular Motility: Theory and Management of Strabismus*. 3rd ed. St. Louis: CV Mosby; 1985.

The preceding texts have contributed to my education in the field of strabismus. In addition, because abnormal retinocalcarine projection may be a cause of concomitant strabismus in otherwise normal subjects, and because it is well known to occur in human albinos, I would reference the following:

Lessell S. Esotropia and anomalous retinocalcarine projections. *Arch Ophthalmol* 1987;105:613.
McCormack GL. Electrophysiologic evidence for normal optic nerve fiber projections in normally pigmented squinters. *Invest Ophthalmol* 1987;14:931–935.
St. John R, Timney B. Interhemispheric transmission delays in the human strabismics. *Hum Neurobiol* 1986;5:97–103.

On these and related topics also see:

Lessell S. Handedness and esotropia. *Arch Ophthalmol* 1986;104:1492–1494.
Lund RD, Mitchell DE, Henry GH. Squint-induced modification of callosal connection in cats. *Brain Res* 1978;144:169–172.

Chapter 5

Hubbard BAF, Karnofsky ES. In: *Plato's Protagorus: A Socratic Commentary*. Chicago: University of Chicago Press; 1984:Book IX, Sect. 51.

For a fuller discussion of my views on the process of classification in medicine and the crucial and central role it plays in the genesis of hypotheses, planning of research, and diagnosis and treatment of patients, see the discussion in Chapter 1.

Silverman WA, Flynn JT, eds. *Retinopathy of Prematurity*. Boston: Blackwell Scientific; 1985:1–18.

Chapter 6

Blake W. *The Marriage of Heaven and Hell*. In: Johnson ML, Grant JE, eds. *Blake's Poetry and Designs*. New York: Norton; 1979:93, Plate 14.

In this chapter, we return to the clinic, to the patient with strabismus and to the world in which that patient lives. The object is to suggest a framework for clinical research within which the predictions of the central hypothesis might be tested. Clinically based research on strabismus is notoriously difficult. The following reading list contains many of the sources I consulted in thinking of experiments that might need to be done on our subjects.

Archer SM, Helveston EM, Miller KK, Ellis FD. Stereopsis in normal infants and infants with congenital esotropia. *Am J Ophthalmol* 1986;101:591–596.
Archer SM, Sondhi N, Helveston EM. Strabismus in infancy. *Ophthalmology* 1989;96:133–137.
Boylan C, Clement RA, Howrie A. Normal visual pathway routing in dissociated vertical deviation. *Invest Ophthalmol Vis Sci* 1988;29:1165–1167.
Ciancia AO. Ocular motor disturbances and VER findings in patients with early monocular loss of vision. *Graefes Arch Clin Exp Ophthalmol* 1988;226:108–110.

Collewijn H, Apkarian P, Spekreijse H. The oculomotor behavior of human albinos. *Brain* 1985;108:1–28.

Eizenman M, Skarf B, McCulloch D. Detection of early development of binocular fusion in infants. ARVO Abstracts. *Invest Ophthalmol Vis Sci* 1988;29(Suppl):25.

Eizenman M, Skarf B, McCulloch D. Development of binocular vision in infants. ARVO Abstracts. *Invest Ophthalmol Vis Sci* 1989;30(Suppl):313.

Fitzgerald BA, Billson FA. Dissociated vertical deviation: Evidence of abnormal visual pathway projection. *Br J Ophthalmol* 1984;68:801–806.

Guyton DL, Allen J, Simons K, Scattergood KD. Remote optical systems for ophthalmic examination and vision research. *Appl Opt* 1987;26:1517–1526.

Guyton DL, Moss A, Simons K. Automated measurement of strabismic deviations using a remote haploscope and an infrared television based eye tracker. *Trans Am Ophthalmol Soc* 1987;85:320–331.

Jampel RS, Fells P. Monocular elevation paresis caused by a central nervous system lesion. *Arch Ophthalmol* 1968;80:45–47.

Kitaoji H, Toyama K. Preservation of position and motion stereopsis in strabismic subjects. *Invest Ophthalmol Vis Sci* 1987;28:1260–1267.

Lessel S. Handedness and esotropia. *Arch Ophthalmol* 1986;104:1492–1494.

Mahendrastari R, Verriest G. Monocular and binocular visual fields in different types of strabismus. *Bull Soc Belg Ophthalmol* 1986;213:77–81.

Mehdorn E. Suppression scotomas in primary microstrabismus – A perimetric artifact. *Doc Ophthalmol* 1989;71:1–18.

Mohindra I, Zwaan J, Held R, Brill S, Zwaan F. Development of acuity and stereopsis in infants with esotropia. *Ophthalmology* 1985;92:691–697.

Nashold BS, Seaber JH. Defects in ocular motility after stereotactic midbrain lesions in man. *Arch Ophthalmol* 1972;88:245–248.

Regal DM. The coordination of eye and head movements during early infancy: A selective review. *Behav Brain Res* 1983;10:125–132.

Robb RM, Rodier DW. The variable clinical characteristics in early infantile esotropia. *J Pediatr Ophthalmol Strabismus* 1987;24:276–281.

Schor C, Bridgeman B, Tyler CW. Spatial characteristics of static and dynamic stereoacuity in strabismus. *Invest Ophthalmol Vis Sci* 1983;24:1572–1579.

Shea SL, Fox R, Aslin RN, Dumais ST. Assessment of stereopsis in human infants. *Invest Ophthalmol Vis Sci* 1980;19:1400–1404.

Sireteanu R. Binocular vision in strabismic humans with alternating fixation. *Vision Res* 1982;22:889–896.

Smith EL, Levi DM, Harwerth RS, White JM. Color vision is altered during the suppression phase of binocular rivalry. *Science* 1982;218:802–804.

Sokol S, Peli E, Moskowitz A, Reese D. Pursuit eye movements in strabismic children. ARVO Abstracts. *Invest Ophthalmol Vis Sci* 1989;30(Suppl):305.

Sondhi N, Archer SM, Helveston EM. Development of normal ocular alignment. *J Pediatr Ophthalmol Strabismus* 1988;25:210–211.

Tychsen L, Lisberger SG. Maldevelopment of visual motion processing in humans who had strabismus with onset in infancy. *Neuroscience* 1986;6:2495–2508.

Walton P, Lisberger S. Binocular misalignment in infancy causes directional asymmetries in pursuit. ARVO Abstracts. *Invest Ophthalmol Vis Sci* 1989;30(Suppl):304.

Wattam-Bell J, Braddick O, Atkinson J, Day J. Measures of infant binocularity in a group at risk for strabismus. *Clin Vision Sci* 1987;1:327–336.

Chapter 7

McKee J. As cited by Teller DY, Movshon JA. Visual development. *Vision Res* 1986;26:1483–1506.

A veritable torrent of literature has accumulated on the subject of visual development, much of it rich in the kind of detail dear to the heart of the specialist. I have chosen to cite only those works that served as a guide for my thinking and as a boundary within which practitioners of the specialty can be expected to operate. The above-cited article is a very special overview of visual development.

Aslin RN, Dumais ST. Binocular vision in infants: A review and theoretical framework. *Adv Child Dev Behav* 1980;15:53–94.

Boothe RG, Dobson V, Teller DY. Postnatal development of vision in human and nonhuman primates. *Annu Rev Neurosci* 1985;8:495–545.

Wilson HR. Development of spatiotemporal mechanisms in infant vision. *Vision Res* 1988;28:611–628.

Wise SP, Desimone R. Behavioral neurophysiology: Insights into seeing and grasping. *Science* 1988;242:736–741.

Modern Techniques of Assessing Infant Vision

I consulted among other sources:

Birch EE, Stager DR. Monocular acuity and stereopsis in infantile esotropia. *Invest Ophthalmol Vis Sci* 1985;26:1624–1630.

Dobson V, D'Antonio JA, Bonvalot K. Grating acuity in early infancy predicts grating acuity at age 1 year in infants with perinatal complications. ARVO Abstracts. *Invest Ophthalmol Vis Sci* 1989;30(Suppl):142.

Drotse PJ, Archer SM, Helveston EM. Quantification of low vision in children. ARVO Abstracts. *Invest Ophthalmol Vis Sci* 1987;28(Suppl):154.

Lewis TL, Maurer D. A short staircase for estimating acuity from preferential looking. ARVO Abstracts. *Invest Ophthalmol Vis Sci* 1986;27(Suppl):76.

Mayer DL, Fulton AB. Preferential looking grating acuities of infants at risk of amblyopia. *Trans Ophthalmol Soc UK* 1985;104:903–911.

Mayer DL, Fulton AB, Hansen RM. Preferential looking acuity obtained with a staircase procedure in pediatric patients. *Invest Ophthalmol Vis Sci* 1982;23:538–543.

Mayer DL, Rodier DW, Fulton AB. Grating acuity differentiates good from poor prognosis for vision in infants with nystagmus. ARVO Abstracts. *Invest Ophthalmol Vis Sci* 1988;29(Suppl):435.

Mohn G, vanHof-van Duin J. Preferential looking acuity in normal and neurologically abnormal infants and pediatric patients. *Doc Ophthalmol Proc Ser* 1986;45:221–229.

Moseley MJ, Fielder AR, Thompson JR, Minshull C, Price D. Grading and recognition acuities of young amblyopes. *Br J Ophthalmol* 1988;72:50–54.

Sprague JB, Stock LA, Connett JE, Bromberg J. Study of chart designs and optotypes for preschool vision screening. *Am Orthop J* 1988;38:18–23.

Teller DY, McDonald MA, Preston K, Sebris SL, Dobson V. Assessment of visual acuity in infants and children: The acuity card procedure. *Dev Med Child Neurol* 1986;28:779–789.

Nascent Motor Behavior of an Infant's Eyes

Atkinson J. Development of optokinetic nystagmus in the human infant and monkey infant: An analogue to development in kittens. In: Freeman RD, ed. *Developmental Neurobiology of Vision*. New York: Plenum Press; 1979:277-287.

Braddick OJ, Atkinson J. Some recent findings on the development of human binocularity: A review. *Behav Brain Res* 1983;10:141-150.

Lynch JA, Aserinsky E. Developmental changes of oculomotor characteristics in infants when awake and in the "active state of sleep." *Behav Brain Res* 1986;20:175-183.

Naegele JR, Held R. The postnatal development of monocular optokinetic mystagmus in infants. *Vision Res* 1982;22:341-346.

Prechtl HF, Nijhuis JG. Eye movements in the human fetus and newborn. *Behav Brain Res* 1983;10:119-124.

Regal DM, Ashmead DH, Salapatek P. The coordination of eye and head movements during early infancy: A selective review. *Behav Brain Res* 1983;10:125-132.

Roucoux A, Culee C, Roucoux M. Development of fixation and pursuit eye movements in human infants. *Behav Brain Res* 1983;10:133-139.

Work with Strabismus and Early Development of Binocular Functions

Archer SM, Helveston EM, Miller KK, Ellis FD. Stereopsis in normal infants and incidence of congenital esotropia. *Am J Ophthalmol* 1986;101:591-596.

Nixon RB, Helveston EM, Miller K, Archer SM, Ellis FD. Incidence of strabismus in neonates. *Am J Ophthalmol* 1985;100:798-801.

Other Technologies for Assessing Visual Acuity in Infants

Norcia AM, Tyler CW. Spatial frequency sweep VEP: Visual acuity during the first year of life. *Vision Res* 1985;25:1399-1408.

Norcia AM, Tyler CW, Hamer RD. High visual contrast sensitivity in the young human infant. *Invest Ophthalmol Vis Sci* 1988;29:44-49.

Chapter 8

Rushton WAH. Visual adaptation. *Proc R Soc [Biol]* 1965;162:20-46.

This chapter represents challenge in terms of references to cite because of the wide diversity and extent of the field beyond the first reference. My approach has been to read widely and eclectically what has been published of late on binocular vision, its qualities, and the control of eye movements subserving these functions. The following sources are among the many that could be cited on these and related topics.

Stereopsis, Hyperacuity, and the "Fine Grain" of Binocular Vision

Barlow HB. Reconstructing the visual image in space and time. *Nature* 1979;279:189-190.

Barlow HB. Visual experience and cortical development. *Nature* 1975;258:199–204.

Blakemore C. Binocular depth perception and the optic chiasm. *Vision Res* 1970; 10:43–47.

Levi DM, Klein SA. Sampling in spatial vision. *Nature* 1986;320:360–362.

Levi DM, Manny RE, Klein SA, Steinman SB. Electrophysiological correlates of hyper-acuity in the human visual cortex. *Nature* 1983;306:468–470.

Mehdorn E. Suppression scotomas in primary microstrabismus—A perimetric artifact. *Doc Ophthalmol* 1989;71:1–18.

Mitchell DE, Blakemore C. Binocular depth perception and the corpus callosum. *Vision Res* 1970;10:49–54.

Watson AB, Ahumada VJ Jr. Model of human visual-motion sensing. *J Opt Soc Am [A]* 1985;82:322–341.

Westheimer G. The spatial grain of the perifoveal visual field. *Vision Res* 1982;22: 157–162.

Westheimer G, McKee SP. Integration regions for visual hyperacuity. *Vision Res* 1977; 17:83–93.

Wilson HR. Responses of spatial mechanisms can explain hyperacuity. *Vision Res* 1986;26:453–469.

Wilson HR. Development of spatiotemporal mechanisms in infant vision. *Vision Res* 1988;28:611–628.

Adaptive Control of Eye Movements

On this topic, which is equally important to the stability and function of the visual sense, I found the following most informative. These articles influenced my thinking on the effect of eye movements and their anomalies on perception. Although not, strictly speaking, related to strabismus, this is nevertheless an important link between perceptual distortion and the role that eye movements play in these distortions.

Clement RA. A comparison of different models of extraocular muscle cooperation. *Ophthalmic Physiol Opt* 1985;5:165–170. [A lucid summary of the state of extraocular muscle plant models, their scope and limits.]

Ebenholtz SM. Properties of adaptive oculomotor control systems and perception. *Acta Psychol* 1986;63:233–246.

Westall CA. Binocular vision: Its influence on the development of visual and postural eye movements. *Ophthalmic Physiol Opt* 1986;6:139–143.

Westheimer G, Mitchell DE. The sensory stimuli for disjunctive eye movements. *Vision Res* 1969;9:749–755. [A gem of an article!]

Other Pertinent Topics

Smith EL III, Levi DM, Manny RE, Harwerth RS, White JM. The relationship between binocular rivalry and strabismic suppression. *Vision Res* 1985;26:80–87. The authors make the important point, often missed or misinterpreted, that binocular rivalry and strabismus suppression are not similar mechanisms. They indicate that these behaviors are different and, in all probability, are mediated by different neural mechanisms. They have to be!

Snow R, Hore J, Vilis T. Adaptation of saccadic and vestibulo-cular systems after extraocular muscle tenectomy. *Invest Ophthalmol Vis Sci* 1985;26:924–931. This work presents the freshest evidence of how the extraocular motor system adapts in well-studied subsystems, the VOR and the saccadic system, to an acute insult. As such it probably touches on some of the mechanisms that the strabismic infant uses to maintain normality, that is, stability in the visual world. The plasticity displayed by the system in the monkey is remarkable.

Tychsen L, Lisberger SG. Visual motion processing for the initiation of smooth-pursuit eye movements in humans. *J Neurophysiol* 1986;56:953–968. This is a comprehensive study of the properties of the motion processing system necessary to initiate pursuit eye movements in normal humans.

Finally of note in the development of the thinking in this chapter are the following works.

Robinson DA. Control of eye movements. In: *Handbook of Physiology: A Critical, Comprehensive Presentation of Physiological Knowledge and Concepts*. Section 1: *The Nervous System*: Bethesda, Md: American Physiological Society; 1981:Vol. 2, Part 2, 1275–1320.

Walls GL. The evolutionary history of eye movements. *Vision Res* 1962;2:69–80.

Chapter 9

St. Augustine. *The Confessions of Saint Augustine*. Translated by Sheed FJ. New York: Sheed and Ward; 1943:Book I, Chap. VIII, 11.

For this chapter, I read almost exclusively texts. I am simply so naive in the field of general infant development that it would be pointless for me to stray far from what is "safe" and freely available in some of the many excellent books in the field. It is, however, obvious even to a novice that the literature is rich, deep, and varied one that I hope in the future will reflect interest in the child with strabismus as a worthwhile subject of study.

Bee HL. *The Developing Child*. 5th ed. New York: Harper & Row; 1989.

Berk LE. *Child Development*. Boston: Allyn & Bacon; 1989.

Fischer KW, Lazerson A. *Human Development: From Conception Through Adolescence*. New York: WH Freeman; 1984.

Illingworth RS. *The Development of the Infant and Young Child: Normal and Abnormal*. 9th ed. Edinburgh/New York: Churchill Livingstone; 1987.

Johnson JH, Goldman J, eds. *Developmental Assessment in Clinical Child Psychology: A Handbook*. New York: Pergamon Press; 1990.

Osofsky JD. *Handbook of Infant Development*. 2nd ed. New York: Wiley; 1987.

Although I did not read each book completely, these books make fascinating reading. Each presents the story of human development in the first year of life from a slightly different aspect (I hesitate to say bias); though there is general agreement on the facts, the interpretations are definitely different. These books enhance the meaning of the process of infant development for the reader and are recommended for anyone about to delve into this area.

In addition, there are several specific references that pertain to the tables in the book.

Knobloch H, Pasamanick B, eds. *Gesell and Amatruda's Developmental Diagnosis: The Evaluation and Management of Normal and Abnormal Neuropsychologic Development in Infancy and Early Childhood.* 3rd ed. Hagerstown, Md: Harper & Row; 1974.

Prechtl H, Beintema D. *The Neurological Examination of the Full Term Newborn Infant.* London: William Heinemann Medical Books; 1964.

Wolff PH. *The Causes, Controls and Organization of Behavior in the Neonate.* New York: International Universities Press; 1966. (*Psychological Issues*, Vol. 5, No. 1, Monograph 17).

Chapter 10

Keats J. Great spirits now on earth are sojourning. In: Stillenger J, ed. *The Poetry of John Keats.* Cambridge, Mass: Belknap Press of Harvard University Press; 1978:67.

Though the topics in this chapter may appear diverse, they are united in the sense that they represent the various techniques for measuring tiny fluctuations in electromagnetic signals produced by brain activity, either under controlled stimulus conditions, such as reading and speaking, or under the influence of environmental factors, such as radiation, magnetic field, and radionuclide infusion. As the literature on these subjects is vast my approach will, of necessity, be narrow. I begin with certain historical references:

Berger H. Über das Elektrenkephalogramm des Menschen. I. Mitteilung. *Arch Psychiatr Nervenkrankh* 1929;87:257–270.

Hounsfield GN. Computerized transverse axial scanning (tomography). I. Description of system. *Br J Radiol* 1973;46:1016–1022.

Radon J. Über die bestimmung von fucktionen durch ihre integralwerte langs gewisser mannigfaltigkeiten. *Sachsisch Gesell Wissen Leipzig Math Physik* 1917;69:262–272. As cited by Croft BY. *Single Photon Emission Computed Tomography.* Chicago: Yearbook Medical Publishers; 1986:8.

Röntgen W. Ueber eine neue Art von Strahlen. *Sitzungsb d Phys-Med Gesellsch Würzburg* 1895:132–141.

Development of the Central Nervous System and Its Features

I found several references in the imaging literature helpful:

Barkovich AJ, Kjos BO. Normal postnatal development of the corpus callosum as demonstrated by MR imaging. *AJNR* 1988;9:487–491.

Barkovich AJ, Kjos BO, Jackson DE Jr, Norman D. Normal maturation of the neonatal and infant brain. MR Imaging at 1.5 T. *Radiology* 1988;166:173–180.

Barkovich AJ, Norman D. Anomalies of the corpus callosum: Correlation with further anomalies of the brain. *AJNR* 1988;9:493–501.

Barkovich AJ, Norman D. MR imaging in schizencephaly. *AJNR* 1988;9:297–302.

Croft BY. *Single Photon Emission Computed Tomography.* Chicago: Yearbook Medical Publishers; 1986.

Fishbein DS, Chrousos GA, DiChiro G, Wayner RE, Patronas NJ, Larson SM. Glucose utilization of visual cortex following extraoccipital interruptions of the visual pathways by tumor. A positron emission tomography study. *J Clin Neuro-ophthalmol* 1987;7:63–68.

Holland BA, Haas DK, Norman D, Brant-Zawadzki M, Newton TH. MRI of normal brain maturation. *AJNR* 1986;7:201–208.

McArdle CB, Richardson CJ, Nicholas DA, Mirfakhraee M, Hayden CK, Amparo EG. Developmental features of the neonatal brain: MR imaging. Part I: Gray-white matter differentiation and myelination. *Radiology* 1987;162:223–229.

McCormack G. Normal retinotopic mapping in human strabismus with anomalous retinal correspondence. *Invest Ophthalmol* 1990;31:559–568.

Phelps ME, Mazziotta JC, Schelbert HR, eds. *Positron Emission Tomography and Autoradiography: Principles and Applications for the Brain and Heart.* New York: Raven Press; 1986.

In the Area of Evoked Potentials

Costa-Ribeiro P, Williamson SJ, Kaufman L. SQUID arrays for simultaneous magnetic measurements: Calibration and source localization performance. *IEEE Trans Biomed Eng* 1988;35:551–560.

Duffy FH, Bartles PH, Burchfiel JL. Significance probability mapping: An aid in the topographic analysis of brain electrical activity. *Electroencephalogr Clin Neurophysiol* 1981;51:455–462.

Duffy FH, Burchfiel JL, Lombroso CT. Brain electrical activity mapping (BEAM): A method for extending the clinical utility of EEG and evoked potential data. *Ann Neurol* 1979;5:309–321.

Duffy FH, McAnulty GB, Schachter SC. Brain electrical activity mapping. In: Geschwind N, Galaburda AM, eds. *Cerebral Dominance: The Biological Foundations.* Cambridge, Mass: Harvard University Press; 1984:53–74.

Hughes JR, Wilson WP. *EEG and Evoked Potentials in Psychiatry and Behavioral Neurology.* Boston: Butterworths; 1983.

Kaufman L, Williamson SJ. The neuromagnetic field. In: Cracco RQ, Bodis-Wollner, eds. New York: Alan R. Liss; 1986:85–98. *Frontiers of Clinical Neuroscience*, Vol. 3: *Evoked Potentials.*

Lopez da Silva. Localizing sources with electrical and magneto EEG. Brain topography. *J Functional Neurol Physiol*, Abstract 11.

Okada YC, Kaufman L, Williamson SJ. The hippocampal formation as a source of the slow endogenous potentials. *Electroencephalogr Clin Neurophysiol* 1983;55:417–426.

Spekreijse H. Localizing sources with scalp electrodes. Brain Topography. *J Functional Neurol Physiol*, Abstract 12.

Watson AB, Barlow HB, Robson JG. What does the eye see best? *Nature* 1983;302:419–422.

Chapter 11

Ramon y Cajal Santiago. *Recollections of My Life.* Translated by Craigie EH, Cano J. Philadelphia: American Philosophical Society; 1937:324–325.

The stimulus to write this chapter was in large part derived from conversations I had with people actively engaged in the fields of neuropathology and neuroanatomy, particularly where these two fields interact in the developing brain. Dr.

Thomas Kemper; Dr. Albert Galaburda, who, though not a neuropathologist, maintains an active interest in the subject through his work on dyslexia and its neuroanatomical correlations; and, of course, Pasco Rakic helped me immeasurably in this difficult area. My reading on the subject has been confined, in addition to the texts mentioned in the bibliography for Chapter 2, to the following:

Peters A, Jones EG, eds. *Cerebral Cortex*. New York: Plenum Press; 1984–1988:Vols. 1–7.

Dyslexia

Morgan WP. *A case of congenital word blindness. Br Med J* 1896;2:1378.
Hinshelwood J. *A case of congenital word blindness*. Br Med J 1904;2:1303–1304.
Kussmaul A. *Word Deafness-Word Blindness*. In: von Zienssen H, ed. *Diseases of the nervous system and disturbances of speech*. Vol 14: *Cyclopedia of the practice of medicine*. Buck AW, Amer Ed, New York: William Wood; 1877: Chap 27, 770–778.

Autoradiography

Grafstein B. Transneuronal transfer of radioactivity in the central nervous system. *Science* 1971;172:177–179.
Leblond CP. Classification of cell populations on the basis of their proliferative behavior. *Natl Cancer Inst Monogr* 1964;14:119–150.
Angevine JB. Time of neuron origin in the hippocampal region. An Autoradiographic study in the mouse. *Exp Neurol* (Suppl) 1965;2:1–70.
Sidman RL. Autoradiographic Methods and Principles for Study of the Nervous System with Thymidine-H^3. In: Nauta WJH, Ebbesson SO, eds. *Contemporary research methods in neuroanatomy*. Berlin: Springer; 1970:252–274.

Chapter 12

Ratliff F. *Mach Bands: Quantitative Studies on Neural Networks in the Retina*. San Francisco: Holden Day; 1965:142.

The thoughts expressed in this last chapter are the product of my efforts to look at the problem of strabismus from the standpoint of as many disciplines as possible. On my journey, I was influenced by many works, but here I cite only three:

Edelman GM. *Topobiology: An Introduction to Molecular Embryology*. New York: Basic Books; 1988.
Churchland PS, Sejnowski TJ. Perspectives on cognitive neuroscience. *Science* 1988;242:741–745.
Marr D. *Vision: A Computational Investigation into the Human Representation and Processing of Visual Information*. San Francisco: WH Freeman, 1982.

Index